AN INTRODUCTION TO
HEALTH ECONOMICS
FOR EASTERN EUROPE AND
THE FORMER SOVIET UNION

AN INTRODUCTION TO HEALTH ECONOMICS FOR EASTERN EUROPE AND THE FORMER SOVIET UNION

Edited by

Sophie Witter *and* Tim Ensor

Centre for Health Economics,
University of York, UK

This book was published with
the support of the *Know How Fund*

JOHN WILEY & SONS
Chichester • New York • Weinheim • Brisbane • Singapore • Toronto

338.433621
I61

Other Wiley Editorial Offices

John Wiley & Sons, Inc., 605 Third Avenue,
New York, NY 10158-0012, USA

VCH Verlagsgesellschaft mbH, Pappelallee 3,
D-69469 Weinheim, Germany

Jacaranda Wiley Ltd, 33 Park Road, Milton,
Queensland 4064, Australia

John Wiley & Sons (Asia) Pte Ltd, 2 Clementi Loop #02-01,
Jin Xing Distripark, Singapore 129809

John Wiley & Sons (Canada) Ltd, 22 Worcester Road,
Rexdale, Ontario M9W 1L1, Canada

Library of Congress Cataloging-in-Publication Data

An introduction to health economics for Eastern Europe and the former
  Soviet Union / edited by Sophie Witter and Tim Ensor.
    p.   cm.
  Includes bibliographical references and index.
  ISBN 0-471-96663-0
  1. Medical economics—Europe, Eastern.   2. Medical economics—
Former Soviet Republics.   I. Witter, Sophie.   II. Ensor, Tim.
RA410.55.E852I58   1997
338.4'33621'0947—dc21
                                                        96–40191
                                                            CIP

British Library Cataloguing in Publication Data

A catalogue record for this book is available from the British Library

ISBN 0-471-96663-0

Typeset in 10/12pt Palatino from author's disks
by Mayhew Typesetting, Rhayader, Powys
Printed and bound from postscript disk in Great Britain
by Biddles Ltd, Guildford and King's Lynn

This book is printed on acid-free paper responsibly manufactured from sustainable forestation,
for which at least two trees are planted for each one used for paper production.

CONTENTS

vi
CONTENTS

CONTRIBUTORS

Tim Ensor is manager of the International Programme at the Centre for Health Economics in York University, UK. He was jointly responsible for establishing a short course in health economics for students from Eastern Europe and the former Soviet Union and has been running it since 1992. The focus of his interests is health financing, especially health insurance, and he has carried out research and consultancies in that area in Eastern Europe, the Baltic states, the former Soviet Union (particularly Central Asia), and other transitional economies such as Vietnam and China.

James Piercy is a Senior Research Fellow at the York Health Economics Consortium, based in York University, which undertakes research and consultancy projects on a wide variety of health issues, in the UK and abroad. He is a health economist with particular interest in hospital efficiency, planning and contracting, the evaluation of pharmaceuticals and the provision of maternity services. Current projects include capacity planning in hospitals in the UK; evaluating primary-led purchasing of maternity care in the UK; and a large-scale study of the pharmaceutical sector in Russia.

Diana Sanderson is a Senior Research Fellow at the York Health Economics Consortium. She was jointly responsible for establishing a short course in health economics for Eastern Europe and the former Soviet Union at the Centre for Health Economics. Her main activities are applying option appraisal techniques to a wide variety of situations within health care, and teaching on health economics and management courses both for UK doctors and managers and visitors from overseas. Developments in mental health and maternity services are of particular interest.

Igor Sheiman was Head of Economics in the Social Services Division of the Institute of World Economy and International Relations, which is part of the Russian Academy of Sciences, and then Senior Health Economist for the USAID-sponsored programme in Russia, which is aiming to reform health financing and management. He is now working for the Know How Fund, Britain's technical assistance programme to the former Soviet bloc countries.

Sophie Witter is Research Fellow at the Centre for Health Economics at York. She is an economist who has worked in the development field and as a manager with non-governmental organisations. Her interests include economic evaluation in health, payment systems and health systems reform. She is currently engaged in teaching on health economics courses for Eastern Europe and the former Soviet Union as well as developing countries students, and in carrying out research and consultancy in those areas.

ACKNOWLEDGEMENTS

We would like to thank the Overseas Development Administration's Know How Fund for a grant which assisted in the production of this book. Colleagues in the Centre for Health Economics who have provided support and advice are also thanked—in particular, Alan Maynard, Brian Ferguson, Nick Freemantle, Linda Whiting and the staff of the information services. Finally, we would like to express our appreciation of the support for this project which we have received from home.

INTRODUCTION

Sophie Witter

Economics has been described as the 'science of scarcity'. It focuses on the three general questions of what to produce, how to produce it and for whom. These questions are of particular relevance to the health sector today, as countries across the world struggle to meet their health demands with limited resources. Health economics as a discipline has become increasingly important as decision-makers grapple with the need for restructuring and prioritisation in the health sector.

Perhaps nowhere in the world is the pace of change as rapid as in the former Soviet Union and Eastern Europe, where the old integrated model of provision of health care has been rejected to various degrees in favour of more competitive approaches. These reform activities raise a host of important questions. What are the priorities for the health sector in that country? What are the advantages and disadvantages of different methods of raising funds for health care? How do we evaluate the impact of different health care activities? How do we regulate the market to cope with market failure such as information asymmetries and uncertainty? What types of incentives for hospitals and doctors are provided by different payment systems? Health economics and the study of health systems in Western countries can provide valuable insights for decision-makers in the former Soviet bloc on these and other questions.

This introduction will describe the scope of health economics as a discipline: what questions does it ask and attempt to answer? It will then go on to describe the structure of the book, which focuses on areas of the discipline of particular relevance to the former Soviet bloc countries today.

An Introduction to Health Economics for Eastern Europe and the Former Soviet Union.
Edited by Sophie Witter and Tim Ensor. © 1997 John Wiley & Sons, Ltd.

WHAT IS HEALTH ECONOMICS?

Health economics can be broken down into a number of areas of enquiry as shown in the figure.

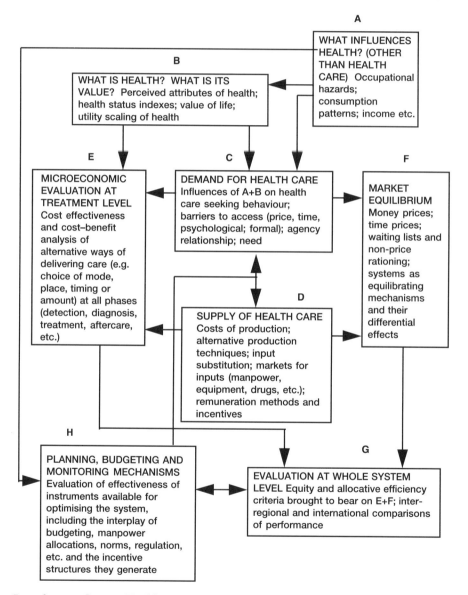

Introductory figure   Health economics: structure of the discipline (Reproduced with permission from Williams, A. (ed.) *Health and economics* © 1987 Macmillan)

In box A come the issues relating to *determinants of health*. It is important to recognise the distinction between health and health care and to investigate the relationship between factors such as income levels, education, social class, physical environment, cultural environment, and consumption or lifestyle patterns and health. Historically, these have been more significant factors for health or ill-health than health care itself, and it follows that intervention outside the health sector may be more cost effective. In the case of the former Soviet Union, for example, external factors like environmental pollution and consumption patterns like alcoholism or poor nutrition are significant determinants of ill-health and must be addressed by non-health as well as health sector activities. An important function of health economics is to draw attention to health gains as the ultimate goal; this goes against the institutional grain for people working in the health sector, who tend to view health care activities as the measure of success, rather than their outcomes.

If we want to make judgements about the allocation of resources between different activities in society, we need to know not only what produces health, but also what the value of that health is. Box B deals with *the nature and value of health*. What does it mean to be healthy? How do we measure the pain and disability of different conditions and compare them with one another? How do we value life itself? These difficult questions require a methodology to ascertain individuals' preferences relating to different health states and to aggregate them into a social weighting (utility scale). This is particularly useful when we look at costs and benefits for individual treatments (box E) and demand for health care (box C).

Health is a good which we value in itself, but the demand for health care is described by economists as a 'derived demand'. We do not value health care in itself, but only as a means towards health itself, or as a response to ill-health, which in itself is unpredictable. Moving from health in general to health care specifically and following an economic framework of supply and demand, box C asks questions about *the demand for health care*. How, for example, do consumers respond to changing prices or waiting times for health care? (This is particularly relevant in situations where prices are being introduced for previously free care, perhaps with simultaneous improvements in quality, as in some countries in the former Soviet bloc.) What is the relationship between what people WANT in terms of health care (subjective desires), what they NEED (judged by an 'expert'), and what they DEMAND (i.e. actually purchase)? And how is their role as consumer influenced by the concentration of knowledge about diagnosis and medical treatments in the minds of doctors, who are both supplier and agent of the customer? The answers to these questions will be very important in influencing how the health market is structured, financed and utilised.

Related to demand is *the supply of health care* (box D). As in any other sector, supply will be influenced by the costs of production, different production techniques, the ability to substitute inputs, and the markets for inputs such as labour, equipment and supplies. It will also be affected by the degree of competition between suppliers, the structure of ownership of health facilities, and payment methods and incentives for providers. This group of issues—the regulation of the market—is particularly important in health, given the supply-led nature of demand, which makes incentives for providers doubly significant.

In most markets, prices adjust so the *markets can reach equilibrium*, meaning that supply is equal to demand and therefore markets 'clear' (i.e. there are no deficits or surpluses of the good). What are the equilibrating mechanisms in the health sector, given that health care is often not charged for, or charged indirectly (e.g. via a third party, such as an insurance company)? This question is the focus of box F. In a free health system, the rationing system is likely to take non-price forms, such as waiting lists, priority treatments and consumer-unfriendly attitudes by professionals. In an insurance market, co-payments, coinsurance and deductibles are some of the options for limiting demand.

Health care, it will be clear by now, is not a perfectly competitive market, in which supply and demand are completely separate, in which prices act as signals of scarcity and rationing agents, in which all considerations are reflected in market signals, and in which the customer has the information and certainty to be able to maximise his or her own utility (or happiness). Supply influences demand through the monopoly of information by the doctor; much of health care is a free good, and publicly financed; and externalities exist in the form of social benefits from disease control and treatment. Consequently, we cannot leave health decisions to the market, but must have information on which to base decisions which will maximise social benefit from health activities.

Box E focuses on one level of evaluation: *evaluation at the micro or treatment level*. As health economists, we are concerned to establish how much benefit we get from individual interventions relative to the resources which are used up in carrying them out. Where interventions achieve exactly the same outcome, they can be compared simply by looking for the least cost option (cost minimisation). Where they achieve the same type of outcome but in different measure, the comparison can be carried out by cost-effectiveness studies (e.g. cost per death averted, or life year saved). This assumes that information about the medical effectiveness of the treatments concerned is available.

If, however, we need to make comparisons between interventions which produce quite different results, then conversion of benefits into a common measure is required. Cost–benefit analysis seeks to value health benefits in monetary terms, which can then be compared with costs to give both a relative and an absolute measure of value (not just whether it is better to do X than Y, but also whether it is worth doing X at all). Given the problems associated with placing a monetary value on health, though, many prefer to carry out cost–utility studies. These are similar to cost-effectiveness studies, but with the difference that a common scale of outcome is created, weighted for differentials in quality of life, by which health interventions with different types of outcome can be compared. A common example is the QALY (quality-adjusted life year). Despite problems in measuring features like 'quality of life', these types of tools offer potentially valuable guidance to decision-makers in allocating resources within the health sector.

Evaluation at the whole system level (box G) is also appropriate and important, especially when structural change is being considered and models are sought from other countries. There are a number of criteria which can be considered here. How effective is a given system at directing resources to the most beneficial health activities (allocative efficiency)? What incentives does it provide to cut the costs of delivering given services (technical efficiency)? What access is there for different groups within the population (equity)? How easy is it to control overall costs (macro-level cost containment)? By applying these criteria to different health systems, we can learn about the typical advantages and disadvantages of different types of funding, purchasing and providing arrangements. These are particularly relevant in times of health systems reform.

However, caution is needed when translating models from one country to another, given the importance of social, cultural and institutional factors and absolute levels of funding in influencing outcomes. Comparative studies reveal successes and failures using apparently similar models in different parts of the world, due to a variety of influential differences. For example, the National Health Service (NHS) in the United Kingdom (UK), prior to the reforms of the 1990s, closely resembled the integrated, state-funded, state-run, 'free' Soviet health service, yet levels of satisfaction of patients varied significantly between the two systems. Why? The lower status of doctors in the USSR and lack of strong professional associations representing them and controlling quality and numbers may be one factor. The low priority given to health in the political bargaining process, and the existence of a two-tier system with higher quality services for the political elite in the USSR would also have played an important role. These historical factors will in turn influence the perceptions of the public today, making certain proposals (e.g. paying doctors by salary) unacceptable in one place while popular in another.

Finally, health economics is also concerned with *planning, budgeting and monitoring mechanisms* (box H) to improve efficiency and effectiveness in health. For example, what are the incentives provided by different budgeting systems? Do they provide the information which planners need in order to monitor performance and improve overall outcomes? What structures are effective in regulating the behaviour of private providers? What are the incentives provided by different institutional arrangements between purchasers and providers? What transaction costs do they generate? The focus here is on finding systems which generate incentives for those who work in them to practice cost-effective medicine (something which was absent to a large extent both in the USSR and the UK).

It is important to stress not only what health economics is and what it can do, but also what its limitations are. It should provide a framework for analysing health activities and deciding on priorities according to explicit criteria, but it is not a complete decision-making tool in itself. Other important factors must be drawn in when decisions are made. For example:

- *Political factors*, relating to distribution of benefits, interests of different groups (e.g. doctors), acceptability of impact on overall economic activity and employment, ideological preferences etc.
- *Cultural and religious factors*, such as the acceptability of certain types of treatments, attitudes towards health, different gender roles etc.
- *Institutional factors*, such as the bureaucratic culture, its ability to run that type of system, collect the relevant detail of information etc.

STRUCTURE OF THE BOOK

This book will not deal with all aspects of health economics, but will focus on those issues which are of the greatest current relevance to reform efforts in Eastern Europe and countries of the former Soviet Union.

The first chapter introduces the main *economic concepts* which are relevant to the health sector. These are important to understand because of the market-based rhetoric which now pervades the health sector. It presents the theory of supply and demand in a competitive market economy and the conditions which are needed for it to produce optimum outcomes for society. These conditions are rarely present in the health sector. A range of measures may therefore be necessary to regulate or manage markets in health. These are discussed briefly in this chapter.

The following chapter (Chapter 2) looks at options for *health sector funding*. This is an area where substantial reforms are taking place in the former Soviet bloc and throughout the world. Given the features of health care identified in Chapter 1, purely private markets in health, using direct fee for service charges, are likely to produce less than optimal results for society as a whole. The alternatives are voluntary health insurance; state funding through general taxation, earmarked payroll taxes, or social insurance; or some combination of the above, as in managed market systems. These options are discussed and the typical advantages and disadvantages of each laid out.

Voluntary health insurance provides incentives for competition between providers but typically leads to problems of coverage for high risk and low income groups, as well as cost escalation where patients and providers have no direct incentive to limit demand. State funding has the advantage that it can pool risks over a larger group and levy contributions on the basis of ability to pay rather than individual risk. Within this category, payroll taxes and social insurance are distinguished from general taxation revenue by the fact that they are specifically earmarked for health. With social insurance, entitlement to services is limited to those who have paid a given amount of contributions, while with earmarked payroll taxes entitlement is based on citizenship. Social insurance is also usually associated with structural changes to the system of disbursement of funds, with the establishment of a third-party insurance agency. This may lead to more competition between providers and to a more focussed role for the Ministry of Health, but it will also increase the costs of running the health service and may lead to fragmentation between regions and a growth in fraudulent behaviour. The issue of designing exemption systems and of increasing coverage in rural areas and the informal sector is also discussed, with practical lessons from countries in the former Soviet bloc.

The next section (Part II) looks at issues raised by the *purchasing of health care*. The reforms which have taken place recently have usually separated this function from that of providing health services (which is discussed in the next section). Despite the importance of their role as planners, priority-setters, regulators and evaluators of health care on behalf of patients, purchasers are often weak and lack the skills and authority to carry out their job effectively. In the former Soviet Union this is partly a historical legacy, resulting from the strong influence which providers had under the integrated system. The two main functions of a purchasing agent are to determine the needs of its customers and to purchase the services which are most effective at meeting those needs at least cost. Chapter 3 deals with assessing the effectiveness and cost effectiveness of interventions, and Chapter 4 with assessing needs and purchasing appropriate services.

The chapter on *economic evaluation* begins with a discussion of medical effectiveness, which must be established if purchasers are to be able to identify the costs and benefits associated with different treatments. It focuses briefly on the question: what constitutes reliable scientific evidence of effectiveness and what are the main issues for health economists to be aware of when using information from medical trials?

There are a number of different ways in which economic evaluation of alternative treatments can be carried out. Where two treatments achieve exactly the same result, a cost-minimisation study can be done, which only looks at costs and concludes in favour of the least cost option. The methods involved are explained, including which costs to include, how to allocate shared costs, how to treat capital items, the use of discounting for future costs (or benefits), the relevance of marginal costs, and testing of results using sensitivity analysis. These techniques are relevant for all types of economic analysis.

Where the outcomes of the treatments being compared are similar in nature but different in volume, a cost-effectiveness study can be carried out, looking at benefits in terms of some natural unit, such as life years gained or deaths averted. The treatment with lowest ratio of costs to benefits will then be preferred. Cost-effectiveness studies are among the most common form of economic evaluation because benefits are relatively easy to calculate if the appropriate medical data are available. This technique does not tell you, however, whether the treatment is worth doing in an absolute rather than relative sense, and does not allow prioritisation between treatments achieving quite different types of results.

For that, cost–benefit or cost–utility analysis is needed. In the first, benefits are converted into a monetary sum, which can be compared directly with costs. The problem lies in the methods which are used to place values on health benefits. Cost–utility avoids that particular issue by using a common standard such as the quality-adjusted life year (QALY). While the need to place monetary values on health benefits is avoided, though, the QALY requires the assessment of quality of life associated with different health states. The various methodologies used to carry this out are explained briefly, and some of the issues arising from them explored. The chapter ends with a consideration of some of the general criticisms of ranking health interventions by any single index.

Chapter 4 looks at *needs assessment and purchasing*. First, how do we define need, and who should make judgements about what is needed by a given individual or population? What sort of information is needed, and who should be consulted in the process? Having considered needs, the chapter then outlines different approaches to setting objectives for purchasers, including setting health status targets, looking for marginal gains, and comparative analysis with other areas. While contracting and monitoring is covered in detail in the provider chapters, Chapter 4 considers the relationship between purchaser and provider in general, and the role of competition not only within the provider market, but also potentially between purchasers. It concludes by emphasising the importance of the purchasing role in realising effective health care and also outlines the difficulties faced by purchasers, not only in obtaining the relevant information but also in resisting political, social and institutional pressures for certain patterns of health care.

The next section (Part III) covers important topics relating to the *provision of health care*. Chapter 5 looks at *methods of paying health providers*, both in primary care and hospitals. Regardless of how funds are raised and whether providers operate in the public or private sector, there are certain typical incentives which payment systems tend to offer. These relate to distribution of providers (in the case of primary care), level and quality of service provided, degree of access for patients, management costs, the balance between preventive and curative work, and the costs of the services themselves. For primary care, the most common payment systems are fee for service, salaries, capitation and target payments. For hospitals, they are unrestricted fee for service; fee for service, but according to some pre-determined price agreement with purchasers; capitation contracts; volume contracts; and fixed annual budgets. There is no one ideal system, but the different advantages and disadvantages can be understood and decisions taken according to local priorities. Moreover, different systems can be combined and adapted so as to constrain features like cost escalation.

The chapter on *provider planning* (Chapter 6) outlines techniques for providers to review their current activities, and develop a strategic plan for future operations, including which services to provide and how to provide them. The next question is how to make the necessary changes to meet that plan. The chapter looks at modelling changes in bed requirements, theatre usage and equipment needs, as well as planning staffing needs, in terms of both numbers and types of different staff, and carrying out costing exercises to predict the effects of changing capacity and activity.

Contracting (Chapter 7) looks at different types of contract, how contracts should be structured, issues relating to pricing and quality control, and the need for information for monitoring and renegotiation of contracts. It discusses the suitability of block contracts, cost and volume contracts and cost per case contracts for different circumstances, and issues such as how activity is measured and what information is needed for different contract types. Although contracting is increasingly a specialist area, the point is made that contracting can start simply and, over time, as management skills are developed, a more elaborate system of specification is likely to emerge in transitional countries.

The chapter on *option appraisal* (Chapter 8) sets out a process for taking decisions about capital investments, going from an examination of objectives and the strategic context, through to the formulation of a comprehensive list of options, reducing this to a shorter list of more feasible options, assessing the costs and benefits of these, and selecting the preferred option. The aim of this disciplined approach to decision-making is to allow consideration of all relevant options, to make explicit the reasons why some are chosen or

rejected, and to provide a benchmark for later comparison of actual performance against expected outcomes.

Chapter 9 looks at the *public/private mix*. It considers the issue of public
ownership versus private ownership of providers and how this might affect
the quality, accessibility and cost of services. This is an important area, given
the assumption of superiority in efficiency which is generally attributed to
private sector bodies. In general, the chapter concludes that it is more the
nature of the regulatory framework within which providers operate which
will determine how they meet these criteria than whether they are public or
private bodies. The role of autonomous units within public services is
investigated, as a potential means to benefit from the advantages of the
private sector, without suffering its disadvantages. The experience of the UK
and Russia is used as material for this discussion.

The last chapter in the book gives an overview of *health reform in Eastern
Europe and the former Soviet Union*. It considers the background to reform—
both the strengths and weaknesses of the Soviet-style health systems—and
then looks at common themes which have emerged during the transition to
market-based systems. A common issue is the search for additional funding
sources, the privatisation of facilities, reform of primary health care and
changes to payment systems, often in the direction of fee for service
payments. Common, too, is the current uncertainty about the role of the state,
and how the different potential roles are to be allocated between health
administrations, insurance funds and providers.

REFERENCES

Williams, A. (1987) Health economics: the cheerful face of a dismal science?, in
    Williams, A. ed. *Health and economics*. London: Macmillan.

Part I

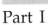

ECONOMIC CONCEPTS

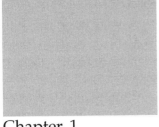

Chapter 1

MICROECONOMICS AND MARKET FAILURE IN HEALTH

Tim Ensor

1.1 INTRODUCTION: WHAT IS ECONOMICS?

The discipline of economics is built upon two immutable facts: that the wants of mankind are considerable, perhaps unlimited, while the resources available to satisfy them are scarce. The study of economics is concerned with ways in which resources are used to satisfy wants. It has been described succinctly as the science of scarcity. At one level economics is simply the study of 'what is'—which goods are produced, what methods are used and to whom are they distributed; this branch of the discipline is known as *positive economics*. Economics is, however, also concerned with 'what should be'. This is known as *normative economics*. Here the starting point is an ethical objective perhaps translated into policy judgements that can be implemented. In this case the task for economic analysis is to show how these objectives can be met in the most efficient way possible. A by-product of this process is that the implications of policy statements are clearly described. Although these implications *may* lead policy-makers to change or adapt policy, the role of the economist is not to dictate what the objectives should be, merely to show the consequences of the policy for the objectives that have been described.

1.2 THE MARKET ECONOMY

An economic system must provide a way of distributing resources so that demands are met. In doing this three practical questions are answered: what goods are produced, how are they produced and to whom are they distributed? There are two distinct competing systems for achieving these goals. The first is that the state should assess the wants of consumers, decide

An Introduction to Health Economics for Eastern Europe and the Former Soviet Union.
Edited by Sophie Witter and Tim Ensor. © 1997 John Wiley & Sons, Ltd.

what is to be produced and how production is to be organised. It then supervises the distribution of the goods to consumers. The alternative, *the free-market approach*, is that the state should allow individuals to decide what is to be produced according to an initial distribution of resources or raw materials. (The state may still have a role in redistributing initial resource endowments between individuals in order to achieve its equity objectives.) In practice, most societies operate economies somewhere between these two extremes.

Three common problems arise with the first, *command economy model*:

1. Considerable resources are used up, often by a privileged bureaucracy, in deciding on what to produce and how to allocate resources to individuals. These resources might have been used instead for individual consumption.
2. Because resources are not necessarily allocated to those that contribute to their production, the system may lack positive incentives to work hard.
3. It is all too easy for the bureaucracy that allocates resources to develop into a self-serving elite, allocating resources to its followers rather than on merit.

For many goods the market mechanism provides an efficient mechanism for allocating resources between individuals. Prices in the market provide information on the relative scarcity of a product while also acting as rationing instruments. Although the market rarely acts perfectly it is often unclear that government could do better and its intervention may sometimes make the situation worse. The debate focuses on which is the lesser of two evils in any given situation: *market failure* or *regulatory failure*.

The first part of this chapter will consider how a free market works in theory. It will be shown that although leaving such a complex process up to multiple firms and households might seem like a recipe for anarchy, under certain assumptions the market mechanism produces the optimal (i.e. best possible) outcome for society. The second part of the chapter will examine what happens when these assumptions break down and, in particular, how far the market mechanism can be used to allocate resources for health and health care.

1.3 A SIMPLE ECONOMY

The first stage in the analysis is to construct a simple representation of an economy (Figure 1.1). Two groups of actors are important: households and firms. Assuming a non-slave economy, all households own their own labour while others own capital and land as well—collectively known as the *factors of production*. Capital can be thought of both as accumulated wealth and also the

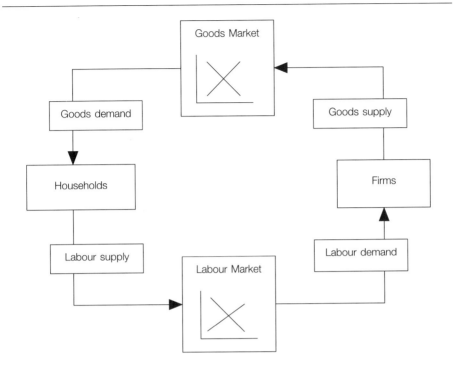

Figure 1.1   Representation of a simple economy

machinery and buildings that are purchased with this wealth. In our simple model only labour will be considered but the analysis is easily extended to other factors. Households trade with each other in markets where a price for what they are trading is set. Sometimes these markets might be single physical entities such as a stock exchange or wholesale meat market. More usually they refer to a large number of different outlets for selling a product which collectively constitute the market for that good.

In the simple model there are two markets: households purchase goods produced by firms in the goods market, and generate income by selling their labour time to firms in the labour market. There are two sides to any market transaction: *demand*, which represents the amount of the product or factor that buyers (firms or households) are willing to purchase at a given price, and *supply*, which represents the amount of a product that the seller is willing to sell at any given price.

There is an important distinction to be made between *demand*, *wants* and *needs*. Need can be described as the amount a consumer requires according to some independent and informed opinion; wants are how much an individual thinks he or she needs; while demand is the amount actually purchased. There may also be a difference between the amount of a good a firm produces and actually supplies. If the price is not high enough then a firm may decide to withhold part of its production as inventories until the price increases again.

1.4   THE DETERMINANTS OF DEMAND

Any description of a mechanism for resource allocation requires a knowledge both of the determinants of supply and demand and the way in which the two interact. In a command economy supply is dictated by government, which also fixes prices. Consumer demand is regulated both by price and by the availability of goods. In a pure market economy supply and demand are determined by individual firms and consumers. Price becomes an instrument both of rationing available goods and signalling relative scarcity.

The economic model of consumer behaviour assumes that the consumer attempts to use his or her income in order to obtain maximum well-being or utility (*consumer as maximiser*) by purchasing a range of goods and services, subject to available income. This may include saving part of their income for future consumption. It assumes that consumers know how best to increase their own welfare and therefore which goods to choose. For many goods this is a reasonable assumption. Information is readily available on their charac-teristics and these can be related to the individual's preferences. For example, an individual knows that rice or fish will satisfy certain nutritional needs while a bicycle or a car will satisfy transport needs. Note that it is not necessary for a consumer to understand how a good, such as a washing machine, actually works—just that it meets certain wants or needs.

For some goods, it is not reasonable to assume that consumers possess the necessary information to make *informed choices*. This is true for much health care but may also be true for other goods such as car or household plumbing repairs. In this case individuals may have to rely on informed agents, who also supply the good, to help make the choices. The problems that may occur in these circumstances will be discussed later in the chapter.

The demand for a good is determined by two groups of variables. One group includes factors specific to the individual that give rise to a specific '*taste*' for the good—for example, age, sex, country culture, family culture, type and level of education and number of dependants. These may explain why, other things being equal, one individual prefers hot spicy food to mild food, or why one prefers ballet and another rock music. Other factors will also determine tastes but are less easy to measure.

The other group are *factors external to the individual* but common to society. These include:

- the price of the good;
- expectations about future price movements;
- the price of other goods (both substitutes and complements);
- the level of development and expectations of society as a whole; and
- the income of the individual.

Although the analysis will concentrate on the effect of this second group of variables, both because they are more easily affected by policy-makers and because they are common to many individuals, factors specific to an individual are likely to be at least as important in determining final demand.

1.5 THE DETERMINANTS OF SUPPLY

In the goods market the supply is determined by the firm. The firm may be owned by a private individual, by shareholders, by the workers (co-operative) or by the state. It is usually assumed that the central objective of the firm is to *maximise profit*, which is the difference between the value of the amount sold and the firm's costs. In fact the firm may have other objectives apart from profit maximisation, particularly if it is state owned. For example, it may seek to generate employment or provide a service to society in excess of the level of production implied by pure profit maximisation.

Objectives other than profit maximisation may be present even in privately owned companies. If ownership is by a large number of shareholders while management is in the hands of a few managers, who may own only a small number of shares themselves, then there are incentives for managers to pursue their own goals such as higher salaries, large expense accounts, luxurious office facilities and attractive secretaries. Although gross mismanagement may lead to them being ousted by shareholders, a moderate level may go unnoticed. Similarly management and even owners may pursue objectives that improve the status of the workforce or the wider community. Although these sometimes lead to increased future profits through a better corporate image and a more productive workforce, the objectives may also be pursued for their own sake to improve social conditions.

The function of the firm is to turn raw materials into the final good or service. It does this by using factors of production: land, labour and capital. For some products the factors of production must be combined in fairly rigid proportions in order to obtain the final product. For example, there is no satisfactory way of laying bricks for a building other than using skilled workmen with trowel and cement—although there are, of course, other more capital-intensive ways of producing a building, such as using reinforced concrete. For most goods, however, the factors of production may be used in varying proportions to produce the final good. Agricultural methods, for example, can vary considerably in different parts of the world depending on the relative scarcity of the factors of production. The production of grain in the USA is highly capital intensive using complex equipment with a minimal labour force. In contrast, crop-growing in China tends to be labour intensive and the level of capital employed rudimentary. Similarly, while the production of textiles in the developed countries is a highly automated process using specialised computer-controlled machinery, production of fabrics in less developed countries relies heavily on a large number of people (usually women) using a spinning wheel and loom.

Considerable opportunities for *substitution of factors* also exist in the production of health care. A modern example is the substitution of capital-intensive minimally invasive surgery using expensive endoscopic equipment for the conventional open operative techniques. This requires training for certain medical staff, including surgeon and theatre nurses, plus heavy investment in technology, which is offset by the reduction in post-operative nursing care.

Economic theory predicts that countries will specialise in those goods that require a high level of the relatively abundant factor of production in that country. As countries develop and labour becomes more expensive, either production methods can change to become more capital intensive, if this is possible, or they can discontinue manufacture and begin producing alternative goods for consumption. This process has been evident in developed countries during the twentieth century. Industries such as textiles have found it difficult to compete with those in newly industrialising countries able to pay much lower wages. Initially this led to a substantial reduction in the size of the industry in developed countries, but later restructuring using computer-controlled machinery enabled the industry to continue with a much reduced workforce.

1.6   SUPPLY AND DEMAND

The two sides of the market are brought together in the supply and demand diagram in Figure 1.2. In a goods market consumers demand products which firms supply. In a labour market, firms demand labour (supplied by individuals) in order to produce goods. In a capital market entrepreneurs demand money, which investors supply or loan. There is no reason why, a priori, demand and supply should be equivalent in any of these markets. In an unregulated market it is the price of the commodity that brings demand and supply into balance or *equilibrium*. This is illustrated in Figure 1.2 which shows total demand and supply at different prices. The demand curve will tend to be downward sloping since consumers will probably be willing to buy more of the commodity as price falls. Conversely, firms will be willing to sell

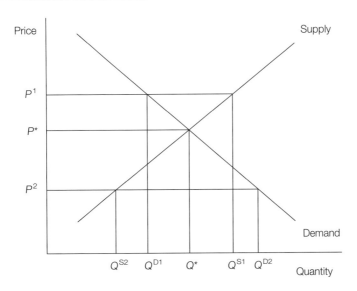

Figure 1.2 Equilibrium supply and demand

more of the commodity as the price rises so that the supply curve will be upward sloping. The price at which demand and supply are equal is known as the equilibrium price, P^*.

The diagram allows us to see what happens if demand and supply are not equal to one another. For example, if the firm decides to produce Q^{S1} units of the commodity, charging P^1, consumers will only be willing to purchase Q^{D1}. Firms are left with stocks of the commodity they would like to sell, at the prevailing price, but cannot (Q^{S1} minus Q^{D1}). This suggests that the price at which the commodity is being marketed is too high and there will be a tendency for the price to fall towards P^*. A similar argument is applicable if the initial price is below the equilibrium at P^2. At this price consumers demand Q^{D2} while firms are only willing to supply Q^{S2}. There is unmet demand (Q^{D2} minus Q^{S2}) with consumers wanting too many goods. In a regulated market where the price is not allowed to rise this may lead to rationing by queuing. In an unregulated market there will be a tendency for the price of the commodity to rise towards the equilibrium price.

The rate at which demand falls as price rises will vary for different goods. The reduction in willingness to pay for a good as price rises will depend on an individual's assessment of whether the good is a *luxury* or *necessity*, which in turn relates to personal circumstances and income. This distinction is, therefore, a relative rather than an absolute one. A man in a desert who is short of water will give up almost anything, even basic foods, in order to obtain enough to sustain his life. In a more prosperous society a much larger number of goods may classed as necessities, such as food, shelter, health care and possibly even cars and books. The economist's definition of luxuries and necessities depends not upon absolute determination of basic needs but upon the slope of the demand curve which will vary across cultures, income levels and individuals.

The extent to which demand decreases in response to a rise in price is called the *price elasticity of demand*. This is defined as the percentage change in quantity demanded as a result of a 1% increase in price. Since demand usually falls the elasticity will be negative but it is conventional to report the absolute value. If the elasticity is greater than one then the good is classed as a luxury, if less than one then it is classed as a necessity.

1.7   THE EFFECT OF OTHER VARIABLES

The model described above can be used to examine the effect of other variables. Changes in these variables can be represented as a shift to the right or to the left of the demand or supply curves. In Figure 1.3, for example, an increase in income, when the price is at the equilibrium level of P^* is represented as a rightwards shift—demand increases—in the demand curve to D^2. The result is that there is excess demand for commodity when only Q^* is produced. Thus the firm can respond by increasing price and quantity until equilibrium is re-established at P^{*2}.

The response to a rise in income need not always be a rise in demand, which may remain the same or decline, represented as a leftwards shift of the demand curve. If the increase in demand is more than proportionate to the increase in income, the good is defined as a *superior good* (this is often the case with health care: as an individual's income rises, he or she may be prepared to spend more on improving his or her health). If it is less than proportionate, it is called a *normal good*. If demand falls as income rises, as with cheap substitutes, the good is defined as an *inferior good*. An example of this, for some individuals, is the demand for potatoes and meat. As income rises, consumers often substitute meat, the superior good, for potatoes, the inferior good. As with the effect of price, however, the categorisation is dependent on individual behaviour rather than objective criteria. Vegetarians, for example, are unlikely to substitute meat for vegetables as incomes rise.

The extent to which demand rises or falls with income is known as the *income elasticity*. This is defined as the proportional change in demand resulting from a 1% increase in income. As with the price elasticity, the impact largely depends on the nature of the good. In some cases a rise in income may lead

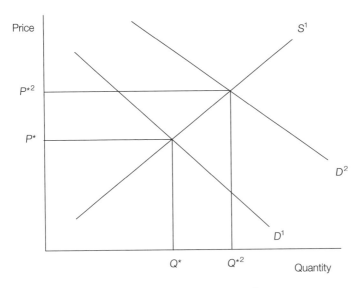

Figure 1.3   Impact of income on demand (normal good)

to an increase in demand. Individuals with rising incomes are able to substitute a more expensive alternative for a cheaper good so that the demand for the former rises.

The effect of changes in the price of other goods can also be considered. For a good that is a *substitute*, an increase in price will lead to an increase in demand. For example, an increase in the price of potatoes might increase the demand for rice since, nutritionally at least, they are quite close substitutes, and the rice is now relatively cheaper. If the two goods considered are *complementary*, so that an individual consumes them together in order to obtain benefit either because of a technical relationship or because of individual taste, then a rise in the price of one leads to a reduction in the demand for both goods. For example, if the price of petroleum rises it is to be expected that the demand for cars will fall. Similarly, if an individual likes milk in tea or coffee, a rise in the price of milk could cause a reduction in demand for tea or coffee.

In a similar way the impact of other variables can be represented as a shift in the demand or supply curves. In doing this it is important to hold all other variables constant so as to isolate the impact of the one variable. Of course in real life this is never possible since many variables change at the same time. For example, observations at two different times may appear to suggest that an increase in the price level increases demand for a commodity. However, if an increase in income also occurred at the same time the increase in demand may be compatible with a *negative price effect* dominated by a *positive income effect*. Although these and other more complicated effects are often difficult to disentangle, the task is simplified by modern econometric techniques.

1.8   ACHIEVING EQUILIBRIUM

The price mechanism suggests a tendency towards equilibrium but it does not suggest the *speed and way in which this equilibrium is achieved*. The speed at which it is feasible to expect price and quantity to adjust to different market circumstances varies widely between markets. In some markets quantity and price can change quickly—a notable example being the market for foreign exchange in Western countries where any shift in the demand or supply for one currency can lead to a rapid movement in the price and amount of currency offered for trading. Similar conditions are possible in the market for company shares, in the inter-bank capital market and in the government bond market.

In other markets, while rapid price movements are possible, quantity responses take rather longer to occur. The market for agricultural produce is one example of this. Because much of the production is perishable, supplier accumulation of stocks is only feasible for short periods of time after which it is in their interest to sell the commodity even if this means selling at below production cost. If the firm finds that it has not produced enough of the commodity all it can do in the short term is to increase price, since an increase in production will take a much longer time to effect (usually a lag of around one year, depending on the crop). The problem the producers face is that they must make a judgement about likely demand a long time before the commodity can be harvested and marketed. If all producers decide to increase production to take advantage of the high demand, this reduces the eventual return to each producer at harvest time. Even if producers take this into account in production decisions, other factors may change such that overall demand is greater or less than anticipated. All these factors mean that the market may never actually reach equilibrium.

1.9   THE LABOUR MARKET

The supply and demand diagrams used to analyse the goods market can also be used to investigate the function of the labour market, this time with the household as supplier and firm as buyer. In a completely free market the wage will adjust so that labour supply equals labour demand and all that wish for a job, at the given wage, can obtain one—there is no *involuntary unemployment*.

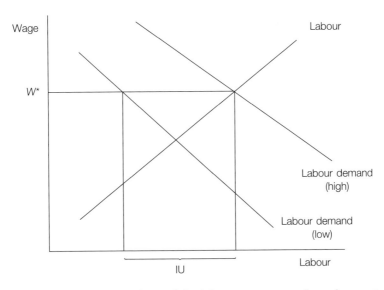

Figure 1.4 Impact of declining demand for labour on wage and employment

A number of factors mean that the price of labour—the wage rate—and the quantity of labour employed may take some time to adjust. Both employers and employees have a vested interest in a reasonably stable labour market. Employers who invest in workers through training may be reluctant to lose workers even when demand for the commodity they produce is low. Employees have an interest to maintain stability of income once employed in order to plan household finances. Both therefore have an interest in reducing uncertainty by agreeing contracts that protect workers from short-run fluctuations in demand. Other factors (collectively termed *'rigidities'* by economists, because they inhibit the smooth adjustment of markets), such as trade union influence, government minimum wage legislation and the inability of employers to monitor productivity, all ensure that the labour market cannot always achieve the equilibrium predicted by economic theory.

These pressures mean that when demand declines the equilibrium wage may take some time to adjust downwards and involuntary unemployment (IU) is observed (see Figure 1.4). This unemployment itself has a negative impact on *aggregate demand* (general demand for goods and services in society) since the income of some households declines. In these circumstances, subsequent wage reductions may even aggravate the problem by reducing the demand for goods still further. In addition, some categories of labour are subject to similar or longer production lags than the ones prevalent in the agricultural sector. Trained workers, particularly professional workers such as doctors and lawyers, take a number of years to 'produce'. A consequence may be that the labour market continually fluctuates between shortage and excess. All these factors may mean, as John Maynard Keynes argued, that it is not possible to leave equilibrium in the labour market and macro-economy purely to market forces, and that government intervention to smooth out the economic cycle is desirable if not always possible.

1.10 THE OPTIMALITY OF THE FREE MARKET

One of the central predictions of economic theory is that, under certain conditions, the market mechanism leads to an optimal allocation of resources (i.e. allocates resources to their most productive and valued use, thus maximising the well-being of society as a whole). These assumptions will now be described.

1. Principal among the conditions for market optimality is that there is *a high degree of competition among suppliers*. This is achieved by ensuring:
    *   *Free entry into the market*: if there is a profit to be made, new firms will enter and reduce profit to each firm to a minimum.
    *   Many firms and households, so that none can individually affect price and all are *price-takers*.
    *   *Perfect knowledge* of all market transactions. This is required for both firms and households so that if a firm charges a price above that charged by other firms households can react to this by purchasing from another firm.
    *   *Equal transport and transaction costs*, so that firms compete on equal terms and households are able to purchase items cheaply and quickly from those firms charging a low price.
    *   *Mobility of the factors of production*, so that firms are able to obtain the necessary land, labour and capital in order to begin or alter production.
    *   A high degree of *homogeneity of the product* being produced, so that products can compete on price and be comparable with one another.
    *   *Constant (or decreasing) returns to scale in production*, meaning that larger producers are not able to produce at lower unit costs than small producers.
2. Another requirement is that *a complete market should exist*, since there are many cases where either a market does not exist at all or functions only partially. If this is the case then there are likely to be costs and/or benefits that are external to the market mechanism that may require some degree of government intervention.
3. It necessary for consumers to have, and be able to understand, *information on prices and other attributes of the good such as quality and effectiveness*. If

this is not the case the consumer may end up buying a product that does not give the capabilities that are required. This point is very important when considering the commodity of health care. It is also assumed that the consumer has *no uncertainty* about their own current and future needs.
4. Finally, it is usually assumed that an *equitable distribution of assets* exists before trading takes place. If this is not the case then there is no guarantee that the resource allocation process will lead to a distribution of benefits that is any better than the initial allocation.

To show how a violation of these conditions distorts the equilibrium it is necessary to return to the supply and demand curve of Figure 1.1. The supply curve represents the price the firm is willing to accept for a given level of output. Assuming that the firm charges the same price for each unit of output, the lowest price the firm will accept will be the cost of producing the last unit of output, i.e. the marginal cost of production. In a competitive market this will also be the highest that can be obtained. The difference between what the firm receives for each unit and the supply curve represents profit—in Figure 1.5 the area *PS* (producer surplus).

The demand curve represents the maximum consumers are willing to pay for each unit of output. The difference between what they are willing to pay and what they actually pay is a measure of net benefit or consumer surplus represented by the area *CS*. Total *welfare surplus* from this good is therefore given by the sum of producer and consumer surpluses.

It is possible to show that any deviation from this equilibrium leads to some loss in overall welfare. For example, in Figure 1.6, if the government prevents the price of the good rising above P^b then firms will not be willing to supply more than Q^b and producer surplus will be restricted to PS^b. Although consumer surplus increases to CS^b it should be clear that there is an overall loss in welfare of T^b, sometimes referred to as a *dead-weight loss*. A government could argue that, since most consumers are generally poor and producers (perhaps a wealthy elite) are rich, the value of the gain in consumer surplus to society exceeds the value of the loss in producer surplus, and therefore that the new position represents a superior equilibrium to that produced by the market place. This argument, however, is based on the assumption that the initial distribution of wealth was inequitable which violates assumption (4) above. A superior arrangement in that case would be for government to redistribute income prior to trading, where possible, and then leave prices unregulated. Sometimes, however, that may not be possible, either politically or practically (e.g. if the taxation system is not sophisticated enough).

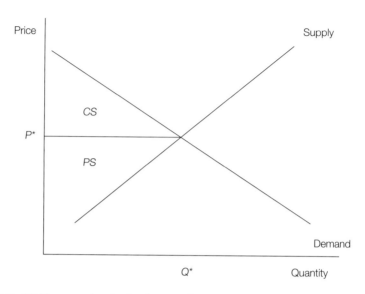

Figure 1.5   Welfare surplus in the free market

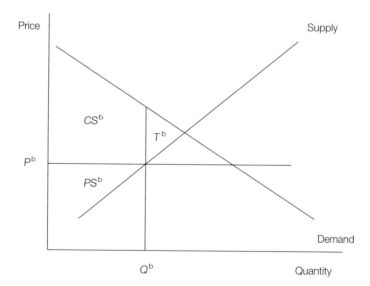

Figure 1.6   Impact of price regulation on welfare surplus

1.11 WHY A FREE MARKET FOR HEALTH CARE MAY NOT FUNCTION PROPERLY

1.11.1 Lack of competition

An important requirement for free markets to operate in an efficient way is for there to be a large number of similar, independent and competing providers that are free to enter or exit the industry quickly and costlessly. This ensures that the product is offered at the most competitive price to users. If firms begin to make excess profits new firms enter to increase quantity available and reduce price. In many industries this requirement does not hold.

- In some the *size of the initial investment* required to begin efficient production—of motor cars, for example—means that new entrants are naturally restricted.
- In other industries the *economies of scale* to be gained from being first into the industry may preclude any further entrants (because unit costs of production decrease as production volume increases, giving the larger firm a competitive advantage over the smaller).
- Another possibility is that firms collude in setting the industry price—a cartel—so effectively acting as one firm (i.e. a *monopoly*, or single seller). Such behaviour is easier if just a small number of firms (*oligopoly*) exist in the industry. The OPEC cartel is the most enduring example of this phenomenon.

In all cases the result is that firms are not price-takers in the market, but can influence price through their production decisions (*price-setters*). Depending on the demand curve, firms wishing to maximise revenue in this situation may choose to restrict production in order to obtain a higher price per unit sold, leading to a consequent loss of welfare for society as a whole (in Figure 1.7, the price is set at P^m by restricting the volume to Q^m, leading to a welfare loss of T^m).

The market for health care is characterised by a number of features which inhibit competition:

- *Some economies of scale (size) and scope (range of services)* exist in the provision of secondary care. Hospitals that offer even a limited range of specialities (general medical and surgical, gynaecology and paediatrics) must generate sufficient demand to keep a number of specialists in employment. Those that provide more extensive services, such as major trauma, require a wide range of support services as well as the presence of other specialities such as orthopaedic departments. The scope for

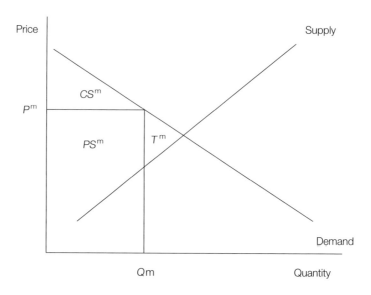

Figure 1.7   The effect of monopoly pricing on equilibrium

economies of scale is, however, sometimes exaggerated and very large units may induce dis-economies through an increasing managerial burden and increasing the travel costs to patients. Nevertheless, the economic and clinical requirements for a minimum hospital size mean that some areas, particularly those that are sparsely populated, will be unable to support more than one or two hospitals. This obviously places a limit on the competition occurring between units and may mean that the market mechanism is unable to function competitively.

• *Restrictions on new entrants* exist in the form of control by professional associations, for example, on the number of doctors allowed to practice, which may be required to ensure that quality standards are met (because of information asymmetries between patient and doctor), but can also have the effect of inflating the prices which those doctors can charge.

• *Factors are usually less than fully mobile in health*, so that markets adjust slowly or are restricted from adjusting at all. For example, it takes a long time to train health workers and their numbers and/or pay may be controlled by some central body, such as the government or a trade union, and so producers are unable to substitute factors at will as market conditions change.

• More importantly, health care is a *notoriously non-homogenous product—* customers cannot simply compare prices; they must also try to assess the appropriateness and quality of the intervention, which it is very hard to do (even for professionals).

1.11.2 Incomplete market

In some markets the costs and benefits derived from producing or consuming a particular good are not restricted to those engaged in trading in that good. This is known as an *externality* and may lead to an incomplete market for the good. Some consumers, for example, benefit by purchasing electricity from a generating company for which a price is paid and both agents are made better off. Other consumers, however, may suffer as a result of the pollution created from power generation for which they are not compensated. The problem occurs because the private costs incurred by firms—raw materials, staffing, capital equipment and buildings—do not correspond to the full cost to society, which also includes the cost of pollution. In these circumstances a number of policy options are possible: the company could be required to restrict power generation to a lower level; they could be forced to compensate individuals/society for the cost of the pollutant; or they could be forced to install equipment that reduces the output of effluent. In some countries the concept of making the polluter pay is beginning to gain some acceptance.

For some medical care a *positive externality* occurs if the benefits of a particular procedure accrue to other individuals in addition to the patient who is treated. The clearest example is vaccination, which provides protection both for those immunised and for those with whom they come into contact (who might have caught the disease from them). These positive externalities are found mostly in public health measures and health education, which is why in most health systems these goods are paid for by the state or at least subsidised. Because benefits accrue to society as well as the individual, the vaccination rate may be less than optimal if left purely to individual purchasing decisions. Figure 1.8 illustrates this situation: here a subsidy is used to increase the quantity of vaccinations provided from the private optimum (Q^*) to the social optimum (Q^c).

Externalities may also arise if one individual's welfare is affected by the suffering of others—a caring externality (also known as *altruism*). In this case richer, healthier or wealthier members of society may be prepared to contribute towards the care of the poor and sick (if, for example, it upsets them to see sick people lying about uncared for in their cities).

Health care in general is often considered to be a *merit good*, meaning that decision-makers are not neutral about how much of it is consumed. Because health care can affect productivity positively and because it can be so important to quality of life, they would in general like all of the population to have access to at least a basic minimum package of health care. In the case of poor families, expenditure on health may have a relatively low priority

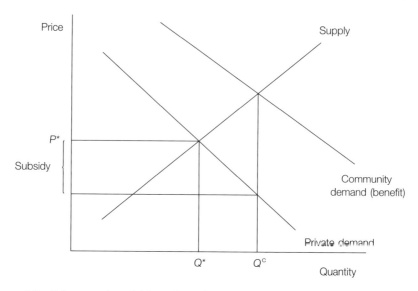

Figure 1.8 Private and social benefit with a positive externality

(relative to food, for example), but rather than leaving it as a private decision, the government will usually take measures to increase access and promote consumption of effective health care.

Some health care goods also come into the category of *public goods*. This is a specific term used by economists to denote goods which are 'non-rival' and 'non-excludable'—that is, goods which you cannot stop people from consuming and whose availability is not affected by the number of people consuming them. Take the examples of clean air or national security. It costs the same to provide national defence whether one person or one million people are benefiting from it (non-rival). Similarly, you cannot exclude somebody from breathing the air, or being defended if they are in the same territory.

An important consequence is the *free-rider problem*: each individual will be unwilling to pay for something from which they cannot be excluded; however valuable the good, they will each try to get other people to pay for a service from which they can in turn benefit for free. The result may be underproduction of an important good. In this situation, it is best for a central authority, such as the government, to determine the appropriate level of the service and charge people through, for example, taxes. There are not many health goods which are non-rival and non-excludable, but a few examples do exist, such as health education activities using television or radio or control of disease vectors.

A complete market is also often missing in terms of *lack of awareness of prices by customers*. If health care is free at the point of delivery or is paid for indirectly through insurance premia, then customers will not 'shop around' for the lowest price and consequently there is little pressure on producers to keep prices down. Instead, they may compete with one another by providing more attractive services, which may in fact lead to price increases rather than reductions (this is referred to as *non-price competition*).

1.11.3   Imperfect and asymmetric information

One of the key assumptions about the optimality of free markets is that individuals have access to information necessary to assess the value of the good they are considering purchasing. In health care markets consumers often do not know what type of care will generate greatest improvements in their health status and must rely on the providers to advise them. As Williams (1987) puts it:

> it is as if we go shopping knowing only that we feel hungry, with not much knowledge as to why we feel hungry, or whether our hunger will go away all by itself in due course, or whether there is anything that can be done to assuage it, and, if so, what the most (cost-) effective way of doing that might be.

Individuals may not even be in a position to evaluate the effectiveness of the treatment once it has occurred since factors such as age and other illness may obscure the impact of treatment. Consumer knowledge and preferences are to a large extent determined by wrong past choices. In health care choices are made less frequently and the consequence of making a wrong choice is potentially more serious. Additionally, the complexity of medical diagnosis and procedures available make obtaining accurate knowledge difficult and costly. After all, if doctors are not certain about the effectiveness of many medical procedures, it is not surprising if patients do not have this information!

The consequence of a lack of information is that most consumers must rely on an informed agent to act as a representative (the *agency relationship*). This agent must have sufficient knowledge of the condition and treatment options available. The agent is usually the physician although other medical staff, such as nurse, pharmacist and dentist (stomatologist) also act as agents. In most cases some treatment will also be provided by the examining physician. The first-level physician, for example, advises on the course of treatment, recommends further consultations, prescribes drugs and diagnostic tests and may carry out minor 'repair work' and surgery. The second-level physician (specialist) examines the patient, provides medical or surgical care and follow-up consultations. The patient's agent is able to influence the amount of health care consumed from what the patient demands without information (D^w) to

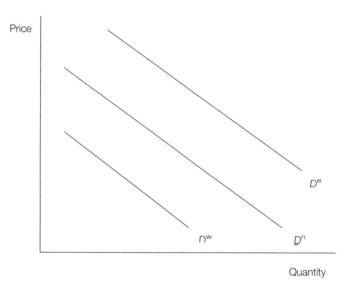

Figure 1.9 Agency effect on the demand for medical care

what a patient actually requires (D^n) or even beyond that level (D^e) (see Figure 1.9).

While some *supplier-induced demand* is necessary, given the patient's lack of information, it also opens the way for possible abuse, particularly if the physician's income is directly linked to the amount of treatment provided or where salaries are so low that staff are willing to trade their own professional ethics for additional income by inducing unnecessary demand. In this situation some government intervention is required to protect patient interests. Common approaches (to be discussed in subsequent chapters) include: regulating the medical profession; altering financial incentives through modified payment systems for doctors; providing additional information for patients; and appointing purchasers to negotiate with medical providers on the patients' behalf.

The demand for health care is also inherently *uncertain*, which violates another condition of free-market optimality. Nobody knows when or how illness is going to strike, and when it does it is often very expensive as well as being critical to the person's well-being. This means that consumers cannot budget for health care in a rational way, as they would for regular purchases, and require some sort of insurance system, collective or private. The existence of insurance markets for health introduce a number of issues, which will be discussed in Chapter 2.

1.11.4   Maldistribution of income

In most societies wealth is distributed unequally, and so is health. Ill-health is often correlated with poverty, due to factors such as poor housing, nutrition and education. This means that market mechanisms will not allocate health care according to greatest need, leading to various interventions to promote *equity*.

In the generalised case described in Section 1.10 it was suggested that equity objectives are better achieved through the tax/benefit system rather than through direct market intervention. While this is true for inequities in wealth, such an approach may not be feasible for health and health care. The uncertain and potentially catastrophic nature of health care demand, together with the difficulty in redistributing income in a way that accurately corresponds to the overall objective of redistributing health, makes some kind of additional government intervention desirable.

In many countries this has led governments to intervene both in the funding and provision of health care. However, although there is certainly some need for government intervention and regulation, this may not mean that it is desirable to dispense with the market mechanism entirely. In certain circumstances it may be desirable and feasible for the government to allocate resources to health care on an individual's behalf while allowing providers to compete with each other to meet this demand. This notion of an internal market is the basis of recent health system reforms in the UK, New Zealand, the Netherlands and parts of Russia. The strengths and weaknesses of such an approach will be considered in later chapters.

1.12   CONCLUSION

Applying a conventional market framework to health markets highlights a number of ways in which markets may fail and government intervention is necessary. On the demand side the two most important are a lack of information available to consumers and a lack of a market for uncertainty. Both these suggest that private unregulated funding of health care may be inefficient and access to health care inequitable. Additionally failure in the tax–benefit system to reallocate wealth and health to achieve equity objectives enhance the need to orient services towards certain disadvantaged groups. On the supply side the presence of considerable monopoly power may render private provision inefficient.

A range of options are available to correct these failings ranging from complete state control over funding and provision, through managed markets now popular in Western Europe, to the loose, and often ineffective, regulation imposed on private health care in the USA. The following chapters will discuss these options in more detail, looking at solutions being employed in Western countries and in the former Soviet bloc.

REFERENCES AND FURTHER READING

Folland, S., Goodman, A.C. & Stano, M. (1993) *The economics of health and health care.* Basingstoke: Macmillan (introductory health economics; relies mainly on US experience).
Mooney, G. (1992) *Economics, medicine and health care.* London: Harvester Wheatsheaf, 2nd edition (basic introduction to health economics).
Samuelson, P. & Nordhaus, W. (latest edition) *Economics.* New York: McGraw-Hill (a general introduction to economics).
Williams, A. (1987) Health economics: the cheerful face of a dismal science?, in Williams, A., ed. *Health and economics.* London: Macmillan.
Wonnacott, P. & Wonnacott, R. (latest edition) *An introduction to microeconomics.* New York: McGraw-Hill (a general introduction to economics).

Part II

FINANCING HEALTH SERVICES

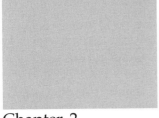

Chapter 2

OPTIONS FOR HEALTH SECTOR FUNDING

Tim Ensor

The last chapter described why a private market for health care where users pay directly for treatment is usually an inefficient and inequitable way of allocating resources. This chapter will consider a range of other options for health sector funding. It will begin by examining the advantages and dis-advantages of relying on private insurance to fund care and will then consider the range of state funding options. Finally, it will discuss ways in which these funding options might be combined through managed markets. It should be noted that the discussion here is largely restricted to the source of funding and not to the way in which money is paid to providers. Although fee for service systems, for example, are often associated with insurance systems while global budgeting is often associated with taxation, this need not be the case. Indeed, many of the reforms taking place in OECD countries have focused on the disbursement of funds without changing the source of funding. This issue is discussed further in Chapter 5.

2.1 WHY INSURE FOR HEALTH CARE?

Since illness is unexpected much potential *demand for health care is uncertain*. This makes it difficult for households to plan their budgets so that income is available at the right time for health care needs. This is true for most acute medical needs and much elective care. Some needs can, however, be pre-dicted: childbirth for many people is a planned choice and preventive treatment such as dental check-ups are obtained on a regular basis. Insurance may not be required for these needs although they may still be provided at zero user cost in order to promote equity or as a response to positive externalities of treatment (as described in the last chapter).

An Introduction to Health Economics for Eastern Europe and the Former Soviet Union.
Edited by Sophie Witter and Tim Ensor. © 1997 John Wiley & Sons, Ltd.

A second reason for insurance is that expenditure required to alleviate ill-health can have *catastrophic consequences for household budgets*. Long stays in hospital, complicated surgical procedures, diagnostic tests and specialist follow-up consultations can be very expensive. This does not apply to all illness. The cost of a consultation with an internist followed by a course of drugs, even if unpredictable, will be within many household budgets, although some will find even small expenditures difficult to pay.

A third reason is that *much illness occurs when individual or household income is low*. Childhood, childbirth and old age all usually entail greater than average health expenditure at a time when individual ability to earn income is low. Similarly, studies have found that those that are without employment are more likely to require medical treatment.

In addition to the role of health insurance in providing a market for reducing uncertainty it may also be used to promote *equity* (which in turn promotes social cohesion) through redistribution from the healthy rich to the unhealthy poor. While the tax–benefit system may go some way to promoting equity in the distribution of income, the health system may go further in attempting to promote equity in the distribution of health itself.

2.2 THE FUNDING AGENDA IN EASTERN EUROPEAN COUNTRIES

Prior to the late 1980s much of the literature on health finance focused on the advantages to developing countries of promoting *social insurance as an inter-mediate step* between piecemeal public systems relying on substantial direct patient contributions and a universal and comprehensive national health system. Developing countries were unlikely to be able to develop their tax systems sufficiently quickly and equitably to provide the services required for a universal system and, as in Western Europe, social insurance offered a way of gradually extending the benefits of free point-of-delivery services to the whole population. Since extension of income taxation was proving difficult in many countries, further taxation increases were likely to come from an increase in goods taxes, which would mainly affect the poor. In this context, 'insurance contributions may be the crucial source of additional finance needed by many developing countries if they are to achieve health for all' (Abel-Smith, 1986).

The agenda in the new democracies of the former Soviet empire is rather different. All already have a universal system predominantly funded by central government from taxes and surpluses from state enterprises. Although funding is low by West European standards, in most cases it is comparable with other middle income countries (varying from around 2.5% in Central

Asia to 3% in Russia, which is similar to middle income country average expenditure on health as a proportion of GNP, but lower than the 8.7% average for established market economies; *World Development Report*, 1993). The main issue, in most countries, is not how to extend free services to the population but how to provide a *stable funding base that encourages a greater emphasis on individual health protection*. The choice that must be made is not between insurance and out-of-pocket payments but between social insurance and funding from general taxation.

2.3   PRIVATE HEALTH INSURANCE

In many countries private insurance companies provide cover for the health care needs of some individuals. Private insurance companies usually operate on the basis that the expected benefits paid out, in the long run, should not exceed the premiums collected for each person insured. If premiums exceed benefits, beyond a basic operating margin, then a profit is made. What happens to the profit depends on the company's basis of operation. Some companies have to show a return to shareholders (joint-stock or share-holding) and the profit is redistributed as dividends. Others redistribute the profit to the insured in the form of lower premiums. If the company also provides health care through its own hospitals then any surplus may be used to improve facilities.

2.3.1   Setting premiums and determining risk

The easiest way to *calculate the level of insurance contribution* is to divide the total expenditure of the health insurance fund by the number of people insured. Total expenditure will include expected payments on direct health care benefits, the administrative cost of the programme and an amount to provide a reserve fund to cover extra large payments. The premium will also include an allowance for profit. This community premium is then charged to all that join the scheme.

$$\text{Community premium} = \frac{\text{expenditure on benefits} + \text{administrative costs} + \text{reserve} + \text{profits}}{\text{number insured}}$$

There will be some high risk individuals that will consume more care than the average, while there will be other low risk ones who will consume less than the average. Two issues arise in relation to this in the context of private (voluntary) insurance.

First, a profit-making firm could earn more by attempting to obtain a higher level of contribution from those in the high risk group so that the premium is related to the expected benefits paid. To some extent an insurance company can ascertain risk by examining past medical history and current lifestyle, testing for relevant risk factors (e.g. blood pressure, smoking) and adjusting for age, sex and race. This *risk rating* is used in setting premiums in other insurance markets such as car and household insurance; however, the distributional consequences will probably be greater in medical markets. The level of car insurance is usually related to the driver's experience and past driving record, which is associated with income in a relatively minor way. In contrast, sickness is strongly associated with low income, making the burden of large insurance premiums for some such as the elderly and unemployed intolerable. In the UK two types of risk rating are common: age rating, where people are placed into premium bands according to age, and experience rating, which takes account of past treatment requirements. The general consequence of risk rating is that for some the premiums will be too high and they will remain uninsured.

The second issue is that even with information on observable risk characteristics the insurer will still know less about the individual's likely need for medical care than the individual. This factor is compounded if an individual attempts to hide unfavourable risk factors. If this ignorance means that the insurance company charges a similar premium to a number of people with quite different expected use patterns, then low risk groups would effectively be subsidising high risk ones. The likely consequence is that the low risk members would leave the scheme, pushing up the premium for those remaining. The insurance company effectively selects only high risk individuals—a problem known as *adverse selection*.

To overcome the problem of adverse selection, companies try to force individuals to reveal risk information by offering different levels of cover for different premiums. For example, two policies could be offered—one that provides 100% cover for $20 per month and another that offers only 90% cover, but for only $12 per month. The first is likely to appeal to those in the high risk category while the low risk individuals may be quite willing to bear the small chance of having to make large out-of-pocket payments in return for a premium that is proportionately smaller.

2.3.2   Limiting demand and cost

A problem common to all types of third-party funding is *moral hazard*, where consumers over-use health care because they do not pay directly for treatment. Although the insurance company can pass on the cost of this excess expenditure through increased contributions, this is spread between all those insured. To counter this problem the insurer may require the patient to share in the cost of treatment. There are a number of ways in which insurance companies may incorporate *cost-sharing* into their policies. One way is for the individual to pay the first fixed amount of any claim—an excess or deductible. Another way is for the individual to pay a proportion of any claim—coinsurance. Finally, the insurance company may place an upper limit on any benefits paid, after which the patient incurs all additional expenditure. In all cases the result is that less than full cover is provided for the insured population. Insurance companies may also offer premium discounts—no-claim bonuses—for an accumulated history of not claiming.

While copayments may be effective in reducing some 'unnecessary' demand, they can also reduce demand for necessary treatment, particularly for those who find the additional copayment burdensome. Demand regulation of this type is therefore a relatively blunt instrument and may prove to be extremely inequitable.

The problem of patient moral hazard is compounded where providers are also given incentives to over-treat patients, through fee for service payment. In this case neither the patient nor the provider has an incentive to contain costs. This problem is widely associated with the US health care system, although many other countries have experienced similar problems recently—notably, the Czech Republic, where expenditure is rising rapidly as a consequence of introducing un-capped health insurance with fee for service payment (50% rise in the first two years, according to Massaro, Nemec & Kalman, 1994). *Supply side measures* are particularly relevant because of the supply-led nature of demand for health care. Many measures have been introduced to try to control the problem. These will be discussed in Chapter 5 on systems for paying providers.

2.3.3   Types of coverage

Since premiums are voluntary and risk rated on an individual basis, entitlement must also be on an individual or small group basis. Private insurers must design policies that are both attractive and profitable. Benefits are quite likely to be defined closely in relation to the scope and choice of medical facilities and type of hotel services covered. Companies will only cover services from which they can make a profit, which will be those services that they can accurately risk rate and will often *exclude services where the expenditure is likely to be high and open ended*. This could include, for example, hospital treatment for major operations and long-term care for chronic degenerative diseases of the elderly. Another type of care that may not be covered is where the need for services can be controlled by the patient—for example, midwifery care. Similarly, services that are required regularly may not be amenable to insurance although a private insurer may be willing to cover preventive care, such as dental check-ups, if this reduces expected future use of curative treatment covered under the policy.

In providing a degree of cover against uncertain medical needs, private insurance offers significant advantages over funding through direct patient payment (user fees). However, the way in which it responds to high risk and imperfect information does not make it a satisfactory method of covering high risk individuals. The key problem is that handling risk in order to attract low risk types and to increase profit means that *affordable cover is often not available* to some of the population while for others it may be available only partially.

An additional problem is that obtaining a *large quantity of information* on risk characteristics is not a costless exercise. The processing of personal data and verifying claims carries a substantial administrative burden that will eventually be passed on to consumers through higher premiums. Consequently, such schemes are also usually costly to operate.

The principal strength of private insurance is in providing top-up plans for those requiring additional health insurance. Even in this case some countries have imposed substantial regulation on the industry to prevent risk rating of individuals, with excessive premiums being charged for people with serious or chronic conditions.

2.4   A TAXONOMY OF STATE FUNDING SYSTEMS FOR HEALTH CARE

The main difference between systems of state funding (either through taxation or insurance) and private insurance is the way in which the premium is determined. First, because it can be introduced as a compulsory scheme, a flat-rate premium can be set without losing contributions from low users. Secondly, although a scheme might have to cover the costs of those enrolled as a whole, there is no need to maximise the surplus for each individual. Both these factors mean that *contributions can be levied on the basis of ability to pay* rather than individual risk.

There are three main options for state funding systems:

- general taxation
- earmarked payroll tax
- social insurance

These systems are often combined to obtain the advantages of each but it is useful to begin by considering each one in its 'pure' form.

Table 2.1 Key features of funding systems

	General tax	Earmarked payroll tax	Social insurance	Private insurance
Are contributions earmarked for the health sector?	No	Yes	Yes	Yes
Are contributions risk rated?	No	No	No	Yes
Do contributions determine entitlement?	No	No	Yes	Yes

The taxonomy shown in Table 2.1 may help to distinguish between funding systems, although a large number of paradigms are possible within each system. Systems are distinguished on the basis of *whether or not contributions are earmarked* (i.e. collected and used for health care only), *how premiums are determined* and the *nature of entitlement*. Entitlement may be taken to refer to non-emergency care: it is assumed that most countries will wish to make emergency provision available whatever the insurance status of the individual.

A system based on private insurance obtains income specifically for health care based on risk-rated contributions. People are covered by the scheme only so long as they pay the premium. Contributions are therefore both earmarked and risk rated, which in turn determines entitlement. At the other extreme, funding from general taxation is obtained from a number of sources including income, profit, value added and customs taxes. Funding is allocated to the health and other sectors by government, and entitlement is universal.

Interest in funding options that exploit features of both these regimes arises from the recognition that risk rating often conflicts with equity objectives but that funding from general taxation is subject to changing political priorities. The distinction between the three public funding options is often not clear and definitions do vary between countries, but in their 'pure' form they might be characterised by differences in entitlement and earmarking. Earmarked payroll funding is where a tax is raised specifically for health but entitlement to services is still universal and so does not depend on contributions. In contrast social insurance may incorporate individual entitlement where the contribution itself generates entitlement to service. The implication is that those who do not make a contribution and are not officially exempt will not be entitled to free point-of-delivery health care.

The distinction between a payroll tax and social insurance is important since many of the alleged advantages of social insurance could be achieved as effectively, and possibly at less cost, through an earmarked payroll tax. The next sections will discuss some of the features and merits of social insurance in relation to general taxation and earmarking.

2.5   EVALUATION OF MAIN PUBLIC FUNDING SYSTEMS

2.5.1   General taxation

The Soviet health care system, in common with a number of systems in liberal Western countries, was funded from the general government budget. In the past the main source was direct fiscal transfers from state enterprises; in the future these will be replaced by other sources of taxation such as value added tax (VAT), profit and income tax. Revenue is collected into a common 'pot' and distributed between sectors according to government priorities.

Funding from general taxation has a number of advantages:

1. Because it makes use of a range of revenue sources a reduction in any one source does not usually have a devastating impact on overall revenue[1].
2. Since one agency collects money on behalf of all government departments, collections tend to be more efficient than if each department collected money independently.
3. Overall control of government expenditure is made easier because the overall budget for government is fixed and obtained from one source.
4. In addition, funding is usually equitable since all forms of income are taxed and taxes are usually *proportional* or *progressive*. This means that they take the same or an increasing proportion of income in tax the higher a person's income.

General taxation also has several disadvantages:

1. Systems based on taxation may not be equitable if they depend heavily on goods taxation. Since these taxes are usually imposed as a proportion of the product price, it follows that a person with lower income will have to pay a larger share of income in tax than a person with higher income. This type of tax is known as a *regressive* tax.
2. Since taxes go into a general fund, citizens are unaware exactly what their contribution will be spent on. This can reduce a person's willingness to pay taxation. This can be a problem in a developed market economy, but is even more problematic in a transition economy where systems for assessing and collecting taxes are as yet undeveloped. It is currently quite easy for a person to avoid taxation and the likelihood that this will happen increases if it is unclear what the money will be spent on.
3. Annual allocations from the general budget are subject to changing political priorities over what is considered more or less important public

---

[1] Unless revenue is heavily dependent on one or two sources. In Turkmenistan, for example, much revenue comes from oil and gas. If the prices of these commodities fall or stocks become uneconomic to extract, then revenues would be affected significantly.

expenditure. For many years the Romanian dictator Ceaușescu chose to allocate little to health care since he considered that people living under Romanian communism must be healthy. Soviet countries have tended to regard the health sector as unproductive and therefore meriting a small allocation.

2.5.2   Earmarked payroll taxes

An alternative to funding based on general taxation is for some or the majority of funding to be obtained from an earmarked payroll tax—that is, a tax on the payroll of enterprises that is allocated exclusively for health care. Payment of the tax confers no additional benefits on payees. Payroll funding is usually thought of as additional to budget funding. It is unrealistic, in most of the former Soviet Union countries, to expect that payroll taxes can contribute all or even the majority of health sector funding.

Payroll taxes are a common way of funding social security entitlements, such as unemployment benefit, in many countries. A 2% payroll tax was used in the early stages of the Romanian reforms to provide additional funding for medicines long before any real debate on social insurance had begun.

An advantage of a payroll tax over taxation is that the money is guaranteed for the health sector although there is a danger that government will cut back its budget allocation to make up for the additional money received from the payroll tax. To some extent health care is taken outside the political arena and given a 'guaranteed' source of funding. It is also argued that if taxes are earmarked people are more willing to pay them.

However, there are a number of disadvantages of a health care payroll tax:

1. Introducing a payroll tax on enterprises makes it more expensive for a firm to hire additional staff—a *tax on employment*. This could exacerbate the impact of economic recession. Firms already shedding employees may have to cut their workforce still further if another tax is imposed on them. This problem is alleviated if the health tax replaces some other payroll tax but then another sector will suffer from reduced funding.
2. Payroll taxes form a *narrower funding base* than general taxation. They are collected from those in waged employment but do not tax other sources of income, such as investment income, earned mainly by wealthier people. They are therefore not as equitable as taxes that tax all forms of income.
3. While payroll taxes are less vulnerable to changing political priorities, they are intrinsically *more vulnerable to the economic cycle*. During recession employment tends to fall and with it the yield from payroll taxes. Taxes that are based on a wider funding base tend to be affected less dramatically.

4. Many former Soviet bloc countries are currently introducing payroll taxes at the same time as economic recession and employment restructuring. Many people are leaving state employment either because they wish to work in the private sector or because their enterprise itself is affected adversely by recession. Collecting through a payroll tax in these circumstances is extremely difficult and the result is that only a small proportion of the revenue expected is likely to be collected.

It is important to note that *those that bear the cost of the payroll tax are not necessarily those that actually make the payment*. Countries have gone to considerable lengths to share the payment of the contribution between employee and employer: some place the whole burden on the employer while others may share the payment with the majority paid by the employer. If the contribution is borne solely or principally by the employer there are five possible responses: employers may reduce profit; increase prices; reduce wages; reduce employment of labour to pay for the tax; or a combination of all the other four. If the contribution is borne mainly by employees they may bear the tax through a fall in disposable income or they may demand additional wages in compensation.

The response in each case will depend on the structure of the labour market. One UK study estimated that 60% of the payroll contribution was actually borne by the employee regardless of who makes the payment. In labour markets where the market is managed by government or trade unions the response to an increased payroll contribution may be to reduce employment of labour rather than a reduction in wages. In the current context of the former Soviet bloc, with high levels of under- and unemployment, the burden of insurance contributions is likely to fall mainly on employees (in Russia, for example, even though under the 1993 Insurance Law contributions for mandatory health insurance of 3.6% of payroll are to be levied from employers only).

2.5.3   Social insurance

Social medical insurance is usually based on an earmarked payroll tax (so all the comments relating to payroll taxes apply equally here) but includes an entitlement to services that is dependent on contributions. In addition, the benefits and access to services are often explicitly stated, although the level of detail is usually less than in a conventional private insurance policy.

An insurance fund is often established separately from the Ministry of Health to manage contributions. This fund usually pays providers but may also be involved in collecting contributions. The danger is that it simply duplicates other tax collection bodies. Many insurance funds find that they can operate more effectively with the assistance of the tax department, although other countries continue to operate a parallel structure.

2.6   COVERING THE POPULATION UNDER AN INSURANCE SYSTEM

The main advantage of social insurance, compared to a payroll tax, is also the main disadvantage. Because entitlement is dependent on contribution, people are given an incentive to contribute to the scheme. But this may also mean that they are left without cover. No matter how diligent a country is in trying to ensure universality by making contributions compulsory and funding socially protected groups through general taxation, it is likely that some people will be excluded from the system.

A system of social insurance requires each citizen to make a contribution unless qualifying for one of the exemption categories in which case contribution is made out of the state budget. Usually exempt categories include: children, elderly, disabled and registered unemployed.

There are three key issues:

- identifying and registering eligible individuals;
- assessing the size of the contribution; and
- collecting the contribution.

Each of these presents distinct problems for the insurance agency. In some areas of a country it may prove difficult to identify those that should contribute. In Mongolia, it has been difficult to identify many of those people in nomadic ethnic groups because they move around so frequently. Once identified, assessment of individuals can also be difficult where individuals work for themselves or have many different forms of employment. Avoiding taxation is a way of life for the majority of people living in transitional economies, and the best that tax or insurance agencies can hope for is to approximate the level of income.

For *assessment* purposes the eligible population might be divided into four groups:

1. Workers in state or large private sector enterprises, and civil servants.
2. Self-employed or workers in small private sector enterprises.
3. Rural workers.
4. Dependants and the unregistered unemployed.

The first group is usually relatively easy to assess since the size of the payroll is easily observable and it requires relatively little effort by collectors to ensure that the entire enterprise is registered. It is reported that in some countries it has actually proved easier to register private sector enterprises since they are often afraid of having their licences revoked if they contravene regulations.

The second group carries with it the international problem of assessing the income of a small business. Many industrialised countries depend to a large extent on self-assessment, supported by sophisticated statistical methods for identifying those businesses that appear to be under-reporting income. Yet these methods do not generally exist in former Soviet Union countries. The confusion about which taxes should be collected nationally and which locally and by whom adds to the problems of effective collection.

Many of the people living in rural areas would originally have worked for state farms and fallen under the state enterprise system. As these farms break up, rural employment becomes more diverse and scattered and collecting contributions much harder. These problems are likely to be worse in countries where the rate of urbanisation is relatively low and where the population is scattered. This suggests problems will be more severe in remoter areas of Russia and large parts of Central Asia and less severe in Eastern Europe and the Baltic Republics. It also means that a different approach to insurance may be required in these countries. Some options are given in section 2.6.1.

The final group are those that are non-working but not entitled to state-subsidised insurance. One group are the wives or husbands of workers employed by enterprises. In many schemes in OECD countries this group would be covered automatically by the work-related insurance, sometimes by the payment of a small additional premium. Another group are those who are not entitled to register as unemployed, because of tight rules about eligibility, but who are still non-working or working in the informal sector (e.g. working on a roadside stall, or driving a private car as a 'taxi').

Many countries have introduced insurance gradually by first covering the first group and then extending coverage to these other groups. While this is often acceptable in developing countries where entitlement to free services has never been universal, in former Soviet Union countries it is much harder to take away entitlement. An alternative is to continue to provide universal entitlement but to introduce insurance as a payroll tax in the first instance. The problem with this is that there is no incentive for other groups to begin contributing. Some of the former Soviet Union countries are setting a time limit on universal entitlement after which entitlement will be based on contributions. It remains to be seen whether this approach will work.

The final problem is to *collect* contributions. This is a particular problem with enterprises struggling to remain in business. Obtaining further contributions from them may prove difficult. The state will have to take the difficult decision whether to obtain the contribution by force, possibly bankrupting the enterprise and putting many people out of work, or waiving the contribution and setting a bad example to other enterprises.

2.6.1 Coverage in rural areas

Covering the rural labour force is, for many countries, one of the greatest challenges in introducing national health insurance. Actual incomes are often easy to conceal through a multiplicity of jobs and subsistence farming. A number of approaches are possible, as detailed below.

2.6.1.1 *Ignoring the rural labour force*

One approach is to ignore the rural labour force—for the foreseeable future—and to continue to provide universal access through a tax-funded system. The problem with this approach is that, unless it is properly funded, the system can quickly become two-tier with those in urban areas, who are frequently better off than their rural counterparts, having access to superior facilities and better quality services.

2.6.1.2 *Voluntary insurance*

Another approach is to introduce voluntary insurance, possibly with a flat-rate contribution for all except the very poor, who are provided with insurance cover (an entitlement card) free of charge. A key problem with this option is that of *adverse selection*: the healthy may be unwilling to subsidise the sick so that the scheme attracts only bad (expensive) risks. This problem may be avoided only by setting the premium at a level that attracts all groups—well below an actuarially determined contribution and one that will require continued subsidy from other sources. The second problem is that there must be an *incentive to join such a scheme* (assuming that a basic free service continues to exist). Equity principles often prevent a scheme discriminating in the level of medical benefits that are provided, but improving non-medical benefits, reducing waiting times for non-urgent procedures or giving greater choice may be acceptable to attract new enrolees.

The type of *non-medical benefits* that are suitable depends upon the country circumstances. In Western Europe voluntary insurance schemes may offer à la carte menus, fax and other business facilities, television and private bathrooms. The new voluntary scheme in Vietnam offers improved hotel facilities: double rooms, ceiling fans and thermos flasks for making tea (Ensor, 1995). The principle, however, is the same in both contexts: attracting enrolment by making the in-patient stay more comfortable without changing the basic medical treatment.

The second approach is to offer some *advantage in queuing or waiting times* to those purchasing voluntary insurance. This may mean, as in the Thai health card scheme, providing fast-track access and special waiting areas for non-emergency out-patient consultations. Where patients have to wait for substantial periods for elective surgery, it may also mean allowing the patient to 'jump the queue' and choose a convenient time for care. This is the main reason for purchasing voluntary insurance in the UK. The danger here is that allowing patients to jump queues, particularly for in-patient care, may alter the impact of the medical treatment itself and lead to a two-tier system. There is a choice to be made between equal access to medical care and encouraging insurance enrolment.

A final method for attracting voluntary enrolees is by giving patients *greater choice* in the specialist or hospital that they are able to attend. A government scheme might restrict patients to a small number of preferred providers with which the commissioning agent has a contract—possibly the local public polyclinic or hospital. Voluntary insurance might permit patients to choose other providers, perhaps because they are nearer to a patient's home or offer more attractive surroundings.

2.6.1.3 Individual income assessment

An assessment of individual or household income in the first instance is likely to be based upon a self-declaration of earnings. Although it is not necessary to check each household, declaration procedures should be designed so that those that are obviously false are spotted immediately (a self-employed large landowner earning a very small income, for example), while a random sample of the rest are also scrutinised. Where possible, procedures should be combined with those used for checking general taxation declarations. Verification of earnings is much more difficult than for those in industrial employment since employees are scattered between many organisations and income obtained from a variety of occupations.

Several approaches are possible to *check declarations*.

Where a large part of earnings are derived from one source, it may be possible to inspect the records of those purchasing the farm produce: the records of a commune co-operative, for example. Another approach in the case where most income is obtained from farming is to impute an expected income to a household on the basis of the size of landholdings and quality of the land. This approach is used in Turkey, for example, to obtain an estimate of expected income for taxation purposes. Problems occur where actual earnings are substantially below expected level because of some exogenous factor, such as household sickness or climatic conditions, although a sophisticated system should be able to allow for such circumstances.

In many countries rural incomes are derived from a multiplicity of sources, of which land earnings represent only a small, but variable, part: some households may generate almost all income from land while others, with similar landholdings, might generate very little. In such circumstances, basing contributions on ability to pay will require a more sophisticated way of imputing expected income to verify declarations: a simple 'crop tax' will vastly underestimate the actual earnings of many households. This violates the principle of *horizontal equity*—that those in self-employment should make similar contributions to those with comparable income in the industrial sector. One method being developed in several countries is to use statistical techniques to relate ownership of observable assets, such as consumer and producer durables, and observable characteristics, such as ratio of economically active members to the total, to income using survey data. This same relationship can then be used to estimate the expected income of a suspect household. Although this approach may provide a useful tool in the future, results do not yet provide an instrument that is sufficiently accurate to be used in the field.

2.6.1.4 Community contributions

A final approach is to collect contributions from the community as a whole. This is possible only where there is a clear administrative level responsible at village or commune level. Communities can be assessed on the basis of their income as a whole and it is then left up to them how they obtain contributions from individual households. Village officials can also be responsible for distributing health insurance cards and deciding on those that should receive free health cards. This system has the advantage that local communities will often be able to gauge the ability to pay of households much better than higher tiers of government. A disadvantage is that contribution waivers may not always be given to those least able to pay: there is considerable scope for corruption and nepotism in the way exemptions are handed out.

2.7 POLITICAL AND ADMINISTRATIVE IMPLICATIONS OF SOCIAL INSURANCE

Even if the economic advantages of social insurance can be contested there may be political advantage obtained by making the funding of health care *largely independent of the normal public expenditure process* and separate from the Ministry of Health. It is worth observing that while there may be good reason for the earmarking and independence of health care expenditures, this argument might also be used for other sectors: why not earmark funding for education, roads, the environment? Although it may be argued that near-universal earmarking is more democratic since people can choose how much money to devote to each sector, it does also reduce the scope for government to shift funding according to changing social priorities.

Two issues are important: the earmarking issue is essentially about preventing short-term and often changing political priorities from having a destabilising effect on health sector funding. The second issue is more subtle, relating to the *competence of the Ministry of Health itself* to act as a modern planning agency and commissioner of health care. These functions have not been carried out fully in the past because of the dominance of funding normatives and line budgeting which removed the imperative to think about the pattern of service provision in relation to health need. In these circumstances two options are possible: either the Ministry can be reformed from within by introducing new working practices and expertise or a completely new agency can be established from scratch with the specific function of allocating funding. The establishment of an insurance fund is an acceptable way of achieving that aim. More positively, devolving power over the day-to-day funding of health care to another agency can allow the Ministry to concentrate on *more strategic issues* including:

- accreditation and monitoring of health care providers;
- evaluation, approval and funding of large capital projects including facility development and large equipment purchases;
- human resource management by influencing numbers in medical school and accreditation of different specialists;
- developing the role and numbers of general practitioners;
- approval of national payment tariffs (if used); and
- continued role in managing and financing tertiary/national units under direct control.

The same issue is replicated at the regional level where, as in Russia, a local fund is established alongside the local health administration. Here it should be recognised that the administration has a crucial role to fulfil in administering certain national programmes—infectious disease control, HIV etc.—planning the development of facilities and ensuring that standards are maintained in facilities. (A discussion of this role follows in Chapter 4 on purchasing.)

A key issue is *how much autonomy* is given to the insurance fund and what rules govern accountability: the greater autonomy given to a fund over day-to-day matters, the stronger should be the lines of accountability over its overall performance and rules of operation. In Russia, as in other countries, the Federal Fund is governed by a council that includes representatives of all concerned ministries. Another mode of operation is to establish the fund as a remote arm of the Ministry of Health, directed by one of the Minster's deputies, but accountable to a board incorporating other ministries and relevant pressure groups such as trade unions and employers.

A related issue concerns the way in which *fund control is devolved to local levels.* This can be achieved in several ways. First, a local branch office can be established to collect contributions, issue cards and make payments to providers while remaining part of the national fund. The second possibility is to establish local funds each responsible for their own operation, contracts and financial integrity. This may run closer to the general trend for greater decentralisation but does raise a number of potential difficulties. Having a number of localised and independent funds increases the possibility of corruption, which may be difficult to monitor and control from the central level. Corruption scandals linked to local autonomy over fund reserves have occurred in several countries, such as Estonia.

Even if fraudulent behaviour is prevented another problem is that the *process of redistribution of funding from rich to poor areas* is made much more difficult where there is strong local control. Forcing funds to give up money obtained from local contributors to redistribute to other areas is much more difficult than if all money automatically went straight to the centre after which it is distributed according to some explicit criteria or formula. Strong local control over funds thus restricts the scope for redistribution—a problem that has arisen in Russia itself, as well as Estonia and Latvia. The latter two countries have both now moved to a system of capitation funding (fixed amounts paid per person per year), but not without strong protest from local funds and claims that the national office was attempting to centralise power once again. Interestingly, Lithuania looks as if it will learn from the experience of its neighbours and introduce a system based on central collection and allocation of funding.

2.8   MANAGED MARKETS APPROACH

It was shown in section 2.3 that the central problem of private insurance was the risk rating of contributions, which leads to inequity in funding and partial coverage. In addition, Chapter 1 discussed the way in which imperfect information about health care renders consumer choice an inadequate mechanism for ensuring efficiency in allocation. Advocates of markets point to the advantages of a competitive private market in getting firms to compete in offering attractive products to consumers. This may be in contrast to a public system where inefficiency and lack of choice is promoted through a lack of competitive pressures. A number of countries have begun to explore how the advantages of a private competitive market might be exploited while at the same time avoiding problems of risk rating and imperfect purchasing through appropriate management.

The *managed market* approach has been pioneered on paper by the Dekker proposals in the Netherlands and Clinton proposals in the USA, and in practice through the fundholding initiative in the UK and health insurance reforms in Russia. This approach has two key characteristics:

1. Individuals or enterprises *choose a private or public insurance company* which acts as an informed purchaser or agent for the individuals enrolled by making contracts with providers.
2. Premiums are paid to the insurance company not by the individual but by a state fund which *collects income-related contribution* from employees and *pays risk-rated contributions* to the insurance companies.

A *basic package of care* is defined that must be provided by insurance companies, who compete to provide this at lowest cost. Variations of this system allow individuals to make flat-rate top-up payments to obtain supplementary cover.

In this system, insurance companies are not allowed to refuse patients joining and are given an age–sex-related premium to compensate for high risk patients. One problem is that age and sex explain only a small part of the variations in risk and there are fears that companies will *discriminate between patients*, without directly refusing enrolment, by offering cover that is attractive to low risk groups but not high risk groups. For example, a firm could offer a package that contracted with good paediatricians and obstetricians but lower quality psychiatrists, thus attracting low risk young families and deterring high cost mentally ill. To avoid this, researchers suggest that premiums should be related to past use as well as age and sex.

Another issue is whether in practice *competition would arise between insurance companies* since the provision of health insurance is a specialist business and in some countries the number of companies capable of providing the service may be quite small.

Even if competition is encouraged, any efficiency gains of competition may be outweighed by the *higher costs* associated with purchasing by a number of small companies rather than one large organisation. These costs fall into four main categories. First, *transaction costs* may be higher since each company will have to negotiate a separate contract with each provider and enforce it through monitoring and evaluation. Secondly, each company will have to maintain its own administration for payment of claims and collection of contributions, *relinquishing any economies of scale*. Thirdly, because providers sell to a number of purchasers they may be able to increase their prices in a way that is not possible when there is only one buyer (*monopsony advantage*). Finally, any insurance company must retain a *reserve* to meet unexpectedly large claims.

Box 2.1 Savings approach to funding health care

An approach which combines competition and choice for patients with full coverage and personal responsibility is being implemented in Singapore and is the subject of much current interest (Ham, 1996). It is founded on *compulsory medical savings accounts*, combined with government subsidies for certain treatments and for low income groups. Tax-exempt payments by workers and employers are made into accounts, which are then used to cover medical expenses over the individual's lifetime.

Unlike insurance systems, the account belongs to the individual and any unused monies can be withdrawn on retirement (as long as a minimum is retained for medical expenses) or passed on to his or her family. *Incentives are therefore created for individuals to stay healthy*, and, if ill-health strikes, to shop around for low-cost providers. On the other hand, if a patient wishes for a higher quality of care, he or she is free to choose and pay for it. Basic treatments are usually subsidised by the government, while the full cost of private treatments must be borne by patients.

Complementary to the Medisave accounts are Medishield and Medifund. Medishield takes contributions from Medisave accounts to offer insurance protection against the costs of catastrophic illness, while Medifund is entirely government funded and provides a safety net for uncovered members of the population. A large emphasis is also placed by the government on health education, healthy lifestyles and disease prevention.

This system is interesting because of its heavy emphasis on personal responsibility and its combination of markets and government regulation. However, it presupposes a culture of individual and family responsibility. It reduces the element of inter-personal equity transfers, and will therefore tend to benefit the better-off members of society more than a solidarity-based system in which all risks are pooled. In the case of Singapore it also benefits from a fast-growing economy. It should be pointed out though, that, with an expenditure of 3% of GDP, Singapore has health indicators to match OECD countries that spend far more.

In addition to Singapore, China is experimenting with introducing personal health accounts, while proposals have been put forward in Uzbekistan and the Czech Republic for similar schemes.

The larger the number of people insured the smaller the proportionate size of this risk pool since variance of the actual distribution of claims declines.

Further discussion of the issues surrounding managed competition will be found in later chapters. It is however important to realise that managed markets in health are a form of new technology, and countries introducing such systems will bear any costs as well as obtain the benefits of any such experimentation.

2.9 USER CHARGES: DIRECT PAYMENT FOR HEALTH CARE

An increasingly common reform made by governments short of revenue has been to permit state facilities to charge patients directly for medical treatment.

Often this legitimises a practice that has been occurring covertly for some time. The arguments put forward in section 2.3.2 in relation to copayments apply also to user charges—namely that charges may discourage people from seeking necessary and effective medical treatment. In the end they could end up costing the system more if a charge prevents a patient seeking early medical treatment but they must subsequently obtain emergency care as a consequence of the delay. They also impose a proportionately greater burden on the poor.

A number of principles should reduce problems occurring from a user charge policy.

1. Charges should not generally be imposed on first contact care, since it is here that the majority of medical problems should be diagnosed and treated without recourse to more expensive treatment.
2. Money generated from charging should largely be retained by the facilities imposing the charges. This is particularly true in rural areas where a little additional revenue could have a significant impact on the available budget.
3. Charges should be imposed on patients for self-referral to secondary and tertiary facilities for non-emergency treatment.
4. Charges should be lower for more effective treatment. In Belgium, for example, pharmaceutical charges are imposed in relation to the (non-) effectiveness of medicines.
5. Charges might be made for patient-preferred providers and additional hotel facilities.
6. An effective system for exempting the poor from charges for priority treatments should be devised. If this is not possible it may be better to restrict the scope of charging to low priority treatments.

A danger is that obtaining income from charging could become a major focus of provider activity, particularly if state funding continues to decline. This is discussed further in the final chapter.

2.10 CONCLUSION

This chapter has provided an overview of the main features of various health financing systems. It has assumed that the way in which money is actually disbursed is largely independent of this choice, even though they are often linked in policy debate. It is clear that there are advantages and disadvantages of any funding system, and the objective of health reform should be to combine the best features of each in the context of the country under consideration. The introduction of health insurance is sometimes seen as something of a panacea in the former Soviet Union and Eastern Europe, but it is clear from the discussion that many of the alleged advantages may prove illusory, while others might be obtained through less radical options. Above all, it is important to separate the rhetoric of certain interest groups (such as doctors hoping for higher pay under a different funding system) from the economic reality of health system reform in a recession-hit economy.

REFERENCES AND FURTHER READING

Abel-Smith B. (1986) Funding health for all—is insurance the answer? *World Health Forum*, vol. 7, pp. 3–11.

Cichon, M. & Normand, C. (1994) Between Beveridge and Bismarck—options for health care financing in central and eastern Europe. *World Health Forum*, vol. 15, pp. 323–328 (additional information about the introduction of social health insurance).

Ensor, T. (1995) Introducing health insurance in Vietnam. *Health Policy and Planning*, vol. 10, no. 2, pp. 154–163.

Ham, C. (1996) Learning from the tigers: stakeholder health care. *The Lancet*, vol. 347, 6 April, pp. 951–953.

Massaro, T., Nemec, J. & Kalman, I. (1994) *Journal of the American Medical Association*, 15 June, vol. 271, no. 23, pp. 1870–1874.

Normand, C. & Weber, A. (1994) *Social health insurance: a guidebook for planning.* Geneva: World Health Organisation (further information about social health insurance).

World Development Report 1993: Investing in health. Washington, DC: World Bank.

Part III

PURCHASING HEALTH SERVICES

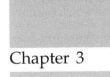

Chapter 3

ECONOMIC EVALUATION OF HEALTH CARE

Tim Ensor and Sophie Witter

3.1 INTRODUCTION

Resources available for health care are, and probably always will be, limited. This applies at all levels of the system; at the national level, local level and in individual facilities and to all countries. Although countries such as Canada and the United States spend a considerable amount on health care, the fast pace of medical progress and ageing populations ensure that the procedures possible exceed resources available. Given the inevitability of the rationing process, it is the task of health planners and managers to ensure that the available resources are used in the most beneficial way possible.

Evaluation of health projects can be divided into three stages: clinical effectiveness, technical efficiency and allocative efficiency (Figure 3.1). Here it is useful to distinguish between inputs (such as staff and drugs), processes (the treatment itself), outputs (a treated patient), and outcomes (the impact on the patient in terms of extended or enhanced life). Clinical evaluation is concerned with whether the process that converts inputs into outputs works. Clinical evaluation is typically sub-divided into two: *efficacy*, where the treatment is tested under 'ideal' laboratory conditions, and *effectiveness*, where the treatment is tested under normal working conditions. Effectiveness will take account of factors such as the poor administration of the treatment by doctors and patients' failure to comply with medical instructions, and so will typically be lower than treatment efficacy. Information on clinical effectiveness represents the lowest level of evaluation before economic evaluation can take place. However, there is still a lack of complete and documented data on the effectiveness of treatments in routine use. One of the functions of the health care purchaser is to use and, where it is lacking to collect, such data in deciding how best to meet the needs of its population.

An Introduction to Health Economics for Eastern Europe and the Former Soviet Union.
Edited by Sophie Witter and Tim Ensor. © 1997 John Wiley & Sons, Ltd.

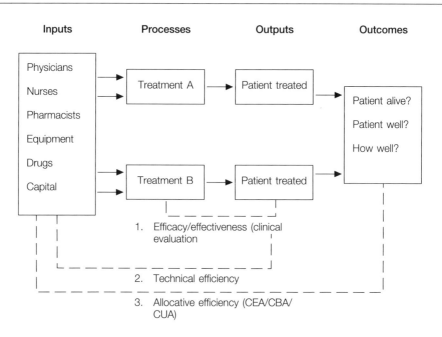

Figure 3.1   Framework for evaluating medical care

The second stage is to evaluate *technical efficiency* and decide which of a number of competing processes for treating a condition should be used. If the methods give essentially the same result, then it may be sufficient simply to choose the cheapest procedure—a *cost-minimisation* analysis. An example of this is whether vaccination should be provided by nurses in the community or centrally at a hospital. If each method has a different impact then a more sophisticated *cost-effectiveness* analysis, that takes account of benefits as well as costs, may be required. For example, if kidney failure is to be treated, is it better to provide continual dialysis for sufferers or, if available, offer them a kidney transplant? In both cases we are essentially interested in how a given condition should be treated in the most cost-effective way possible.

The third stage is to compare the outcomes from treating a range of conditions (each using the most efficient process) to decide how best limited resources should be spent. For example, should more or fewer resources be devoted to palliative cancer care compared to the treatment of kidney failure. The optimisation of this choice is described as *allocative efficiency*. If the treatments to be compared produce essentially the same results—lives saved for example—then a cost-effectiveness analysis will suffice. If, however, the outputs are different and have a number of dimensions then a more sophisticated *cost–benefit* or *cost–utility* analysis must be performed. Each of these techniques will be now explained.

3.2   MEDICAL EFFECTIVENESS

It is often assumed that we know how effective different medical procedures are. In practice, though, many activities are routinely carried out by doctors which have not been fully tested for clinical effectiveness, or where they have been, the information is poorly disseminated and understood. That this is so is illustrated by the wide variations in procedures carried out by doctors with roughly similar patient populations. In the UK, for example, the number of hysterectomies carried out per 10 000 population (age and sex adjusted) can vary between districts by roughly 100% (7.5 in low districts; 15 in high), while tonsillectomy and haemorrhoidectomy were found to vary almost fourfold (Drummond & Maynard, 1993).

The aim of collecting evidence of effectiveness is threefold:

- to ensure that treatments work, and do more good than harm (protect the interests of individual patients treated);
- to increase technical efficiency (so that doctors—or other health professionals—carry out the treatment which uses least resources to achieve the same goal); and
- to increase allocative efficiency (so that doctors treat conditions which provide more health gains for the same amount of resources expended).

If the importance of collecting this information is so clear, why has it not been collected? The answer lies largely in the conditions which must be met to gain reliable results in a clinical trial. The ideal clinical test format is the *randomised controlled trial* (RCT). Its main features are that:

- Patients are identified according to strict *eligibility criteria*, relating to features like age, sex and severity of disease.
- Patients are *randomly allocated* to the treatment or comparison groups, in order that biases (both those that are known and unknown) are distributed evenly between the groups. In theory, RCTs enable the comparison of the effects of receiving or not receiving an intervention 'everything else being equal' and thus the attribution of effects to interventions.
- The *assessors of results are unaware* of which group the patients belong to, so that their assessment is not influenced by their expectations about outcomes.

Sometimes is it hard to meet these conditions:

- Patients may not be willing to be randomly allocated between treatment groups. In the case of testing the safety of home births versus hospital deliveries in the UK, for example, it was found that most women had a strong preference for one or the other option. It was therefore hard to recruit an adequate sample of participants for the study.

- Given the complex procedures and the need for a large enough sample to give reliable results, RCTs can be difficult to organise and expensive. They are mainly used for pharmaceuticals, where they are required for licensing products.
- Although in principle RCTs are likely to provide the best estimates of the effectiveness of interventions, in practice many potential challenges to the design may undermine the results. For example, *contamination* (in which the control group receives the active intervention), *selection bias* (in which random allocation is corrupted), or *detection bias* (in which outcomes of interest are located more frequently in one group than another) may all lead to misleading results.

Where an RCT is not possible, the next best study might be a *non-randomised control trial*. In such a study, the allocation of patients for treatment is not controlled by the researcher, and so there will always be a risk of invisible bias, although some more obvious biases (such as severity of illness) may be controlled for.

Next best after the controlled study is the *observational study*, with prospective choice of cases (i.e. choosing which patients to follow in advance and then documenting their case over a period of time). This is more reliable than studies which rely on retrospective (backward-looking) identification of patients, which increases the likelihood of selection bias based on outcome or some other factor.

In practice, *clinician experience* (expert opinion) is often used as the main guide to effectiveness. However, it is unreliable for a number of reasons:

- clinicians will remember some cases more than others in a way that may bias their conclusions;
- they may have some personal interest in the outcome, such as a belief in a certain technology;
- they will not know whether the patient would have got better anyway or whether the patient's response was due to some factor other than the main treatment itself;
- they may be biased in which treatments they provide to patients with different characteristics;
- their relationship with the patient may influence the outcome; and
- the sample size which they see may be relatively small.

Given the number of trials carried out looking at similar interventions, there is a focus at present among health academics in the West on carrying out *systematic reviews* of all relevant studies and disseminating these results more effectively to decision-makers via bulletins and databases (see Box 3.2). Particularly where sizes of effects are very small, it can be valuable to pool

Box 3.1 Presenting information on efficacy of a given intervention (Adapted from Stevens & Raftery, 1994)

The US Preventive Services Task Force have developed a system for summarising information on efficacy, using one axis to relate the direction of the evidence, and the other to reflect the reliability of the information on which this judgement is made.

Strength of recommendation

A   There is good evidence to support the use of the procedure
B   There is fair evidence to support the use of the procedure
C   There is little evidence to support the use of the procedure
D   There is fair evidence to reject the procedure
E   There is good evidence to reject the procedure

Quality of evidence

I   Based on at least one properly randomised controlled trial
II-1   Well-designed controlled trial without randomisation
II-2   Well-designed cohort or case-controlled analytic studies, preferably from more than one research group
II-3   Multiple-timed series with or without intervention, or dramatic results in uncontrolled experiments
III   Opinions of respected authorities based on clinical experience, descriptive studies or expert committees
IV   Evidence inadequate due to problems of methodology or conflict in evidence

results from different RCTs using statistical techniques in order to provide more precise measures of effectiveness. These are known as *meta-analyses.*

There is also an impetus to develop 'pragmatic trials' which are conducted in conditions more closely linked to the actual delivery of health services, thus making the results more realistic.

Much of the work in this area in the UK is motivated by the new purchasing culture and the erosion of some of the clinical autonomy which hospital consultants used to enjoy. However, further research is needed into effective forms of co-operation between economists, researchers, health purchasers, managers and doctors. One example of a potentially useful form of cooperation is the development of *treatment protocols* based on best medical practice and national models, produced by local consultants and general practitioners for management of specific conditions, such as asthma. These aim to improve co-ordination between health professionals and to involve the patient in the management of their condition.

The extent to which results gained in one country will be valid for another will depend on the nature of the treatment and the way in which it is delivered locally. It should also be noted that most RCTs have strict eligibility

---

Box 3.2   On-line access to medical trials and economic evaluations

There are a number of different sources of information on medical effectiveness trials and economic evaluations which are available on-line and should therefore be easy to access internationally.

The Cochrane Database of Systematic Reviews is one of the main sources of information, containing reviews of studies and protocols for treatment of many disease groups. Subscriptions on CD-ROM or 3½ inch disk for Windows can be obtained from the BMJ Publishing Group in London (tel. 44 171 387 4499). The Cochrane Library also includes a database reviewing the methodology of preparing systematic reviews and a bibliography of over 100 000 controlled trials, as well as the York DARE database detailed below.

Structured abstracts of systematic reviews can be accessed at no cost on the Database of Abstracts of Reviews of Effectiveness (DARE), produced by the Centre for Reviews and Dissemination at York. Abstracts of published economic evaluations can be found on the NHS Economic Evaluation Database, also produced by CRD. For details of how to log on, using the Internet, the World Wide Web pages, or dialling direct with a modem, please request a user guide from the Information Service at CRD, University of York.

A UK-based economic evaluation discussion group can also be joined without subscription for people with enquiries or information to share in this area, via health-econeval@mailbase.ac.uk. The web pages of organisations on the WWW can also provide useful information; the WHO page (http://www.who.ch) for example, can be searched using keywords to get summaries from recent publications, seminars etc.

International hosts like Datastar and Dialog also provide access to electronic databases such as Medline and many others, although these are charged at commercial rates. Alternatively, databases can be purchased on CD-ROM for local use. Contact Knight-Ridder Information in London (tel. 44 171 930 5503) for further information.

---

criteria for patients (based on age, sex, or disease severity), and these will limit the applicability of results to patients in other categories.

For more details on this complicated and rapidly developing topic, see Sheldon, Song & Davey Smith (1993).

3.3   COST-MINIMISATION ANALYSIS AND TREATMENT OF COSTS IN GENERAL

Once evidence of effectiveness is established, the next stage is to consider the costs of the intervention.

Cost minimisation assumes that the outputs of the treatments or processes being considered are the same, and so focuses on finding the cheapest way of treating the condition. This task can be divided into a number of stages: first, identifying which costs to include; next, allocating all appropriate costs to each treatment; and finally, taking account of the time-span over which they are incurred and other adjustments.

3.3.1   Which costs?

Economic analysis generally tries to take a broad perspective of the costs and benefits of any activity. In considering the costs of carrying out breast screening, for example, economists will want to know not only costs incurred by one particular department of the hospital, but also the costs to the health system as a whole (training, support, supervision etc.); in addition they should consider the costs to patients (e.g. travel time, leave from work, anxiety about results, pain of treatment etc., as appropriate) as well as their families and society as a whole.

Costs and benefits can be divided into three categories:

- *direct* (i.e. actually paid, either by the health service—such as salaries—or by the patients—such as fees for drugs);
- *indirect* (i.e. not actually paid, but where a material *opportunity cost* arises, such as losing leisure or production time in order to undergo the treatment); and
- *intangible* (i.e. suffering, pain, anxiety).

The first category will be the easiest to estimate, given that it is based on market prices for inputs (staff, materials, equipment etc.). The second (production losses or gains) involves the estimation of *shadow prices*—for example, using the prevailing hourly wage as a proxy for the value of production time lost. (However, this may need to be adjusted if the wage rates are grossly distorted, or if there is substantial unemployment, meaning that it is easy to substitute for lost production time with some of the excess labour force. This would reduce the value of production time gains made through health interventions.)

The third group is the most difficult to estimate, as it involves putting a monetary figure on the subjective feelings and values, which will vary between different groups. This will be discussed further in section 3.5 on cost–benefit analysis, where the same problem occurs with the valuation of benefits.

Because of the difficulties of getting full information, and because there is commonly a narrow focus on the health service, economic analyses often omit some of the broader costs of an intervention. Where this is the case, studies should be explicit about the perspective which they are adopting.

The issue also arises of whether to focus on *average costs* or *marginal costs* when carrying out a costing study. The average cost is simply the total cost divided by the number of units of treatment. By contrast, marginal costs divide costs into *fixed* and *variable*. Fixed costs are ones which do not change with changes in the volume of activity—for example, a piece of equipment with excess capacity, which can be used to increase treatments up to a certain level, when additional equipment must be purchased. Variable costs, on the other hand, are linked closely to volume—drugs and supplies are the most common example. Salaries are often referred to as *semi-variable* costs; in theory they should be related to the volume of work, but in practice it can be hard to change staffing levels, particularly in the downward direction, and so in the short term they can be regarded as fixed.

Where the decision being considered is to increase or decrease a service, rather than to establish or abolish it altogether, then the relevant costs are the marginal ones. If fixed costs form a large part of total costs, then the marginal costs of increasing the level of activity (i.e. the flexible costs) may be relatively small. Looking at average costs in this situation would produce misleading conclusions.

3.3.2   Cost allocation

Costs can be divided into two types: *recurrent costs* that are incurred annually (or each accounting period) and *capital costs* that are incurred only once or less than annually. Capital costs include items such as initial training, equipment and construction of buildings. Recurrent costs include staffing, supplies and maintenance of equipment and buildings.

Some items will be used for other things apart from delivery of the treatment being evaluated. This is particularly true of capital items such as vehicles and buildings but it may also be true of staffing. To allocate all of the costs of these shared items to just one treatment would inflate the overall cost per treatment and may lead to an incorrect decision. It is therefore important to allocate the cost according to the proportionate use made of the item by the treatment being evaluated.

The way in which expenditures are allocated varies according to the type of item (see Table 3.1). For some items, notably drugs and other supplies, it may be possible to accurately determine the attributable cost. For other items rough rules will be sufficiently accurate. For example, the cost of buildings could be allocated according to the amount of space used for the activity and for what time period. This also applies to recurrent overhead (fixed) costs such as heating and lighting. Vehicle costs can be allocated according to distance travelled for the programme, as a proportion of total distance covered for all programmes. Recurrent maintenance of capital items can be allocated on a similar basis. For shared supplies, if exact apportioning is not possible, allocation can be made on the basis of volume or weight. Staffing costs could be allocated on the basis of time spent on the activity. Alternatively, if this is difficult to determine, the number of patients seen with the

Table 3.1 Dimensions used for allocating costs

Input	Dimension determining cost
Vehicles	Distance travellved/Time used
Equipment	Time used
Building space	Time used/Space used
Personnel	Time worked
Supplies	Weight/Volume
Vehicle operation and maintenance	Distance travelled/Time used
Building operation and maintenance	Time used/Space used
Other inputs	Miscellaneous

condition being treated, as a proportion of the total being treated, will provide a rough guide. Central administration might be allocated according to the number of patients or the amount of facility space used.

3.3.2.1 Vaccination example: part 1

Let us assume that you have been asked to evaluate the effectiveness of a polyclinic-based vaccination scheme, compared to a community-based campaign. The polyclinic-based approach uses part of the existing facilities and staff time. The community scheme uses a vehicle bought specially for the purpose and health workers whose time is completely taken up with vaccinations. We can assume that all the costs of the community scheme are attributable to the vaccination campaign. There are a large number of activities that go on in a polyclinic. Some of the items can be directly attributed to the activity, 100% allocation, while others require an allocation based on the rules described above. The annual costs (in dollars) for the polyclinic campaign are given in Table 3.2.

It is assumed that three clinics of two hours duration are held each week in the polyclinic. The normal working day is eight hours (five days a week) and the clinic space is used for other out-patient consultations the rest of the time. The clinic takes up 10% of the overall space available. The allocation factor for buildings and recurrent items, with the exception of personnel and vaccines, is therefore:

$$\frac{\text{Clinic duration} \times \text{number of clinics} \times \text{percentage of space}}{\text{Total hours open} \times \text{total days open per week}} = \frac{2 \times 3 \times 10\%}{5 \times 8} = 1.5\%$$

Staffing is allocated according to the amount of time spent on the campaign. The costs of the vaccines and the cold storage unit are directly attributable to the campaign. It is assumed that 200 vaccinations are completed each month.

Table 3.2 Costs for polyclinic-based vaccination campaign

Input	Allocation method	Allocation (%)	Cost	Allocated cost
Capital				
Building	Space/time	1.50	30 000	450
Cold storage	Not shared	100	2 000	2 000
Recurrent				
Staff	Time worked	25	12 000	3 000
Vaccines (0.05 per child)	Not shared	100	120	120
Other recurrent (maintenance, laundry etc.)	Space/time	1.50	33 333	500
Total recurrent				3 620

3.3.3 Treatment of time

Most capital items have a life of longer than one year. To work out the annual cost of capital items will therefore require this cost to be *annuitised*. It is not, however, sufficient simply to divide the capital cost by the expected life of the item. To see why this is so requires consideration of general issues relating to *individual and society time preference*.

Consider the following question. If you were offered the choice between one dollar (or rouble or any other unit of currency) today or one dollar in a year's time, which would you choose? Most people when faced with this question would choose the dollar today. A number of reasons are commonly given for this.

- *Inflation*: general price rises will mean that the dollar in a year's time will be worth less than it is today.
- *Uncertainty*: life is inherently uncertain. Banks go bankrupt, property gets stolen and people die. Better to have the dollar now than risk the possibility that one or more of these factors will conspire to cheat us of the benefits of the dollar in a year's time.

But even if the dollar in a year's time is certain and we live in a utopia of zero inflation, most people would still prefer the dollar now because of:

- *Investment opportunities*: one reason is that individual investment opportunities may make the dollar now worth more tomorrow.
- *Diminishing marginal utility*: it is commonly assumed that society will get richer, and as you get richer, each extra unit of money is worth slightly less—hence one dollar today in a poorer society is worth more than the same dollar in a richer one next year.

- *Pure time preference*: most people are inherently impatient. They would prefer to enjoy the benefits of having, and spending, the dollar now rather than have to wait a year.

Now imagine that you were asked to forego a dollar now in return for its value plus a return (interest payment) in a year's time. What return would you seek? Assume that the interest rate on offer was 10% and your required percentage return, incorporating the factors described above, was 12%, you would not give up your dollar. On the other hand, if your required percentage return were only 8%, you would lend your dollar. The bank interest rate for borrowers can therefore be viewed as one measure of the rate of return that society as a whole demands for giving up a dollar for one period.

If an individual saves one dollar, and the interest rate is 10%, in a year's time it will be worth 1.1 dollars. For an interest rate of r, after one year it will be worth $(1+r) \times$ capital, while in two periods' time it will be worth $(1+r) \times (1+r)$, or $(1+r)^2$. In 10 periods' time, it will be worth $(1+r)^{10}$. This process is known as *compounding*.

Conversely, we can ask the question, how much would one dollar paid in one year's time be worth today. The answer, the reverse of the result above, is one dollar divided by $1+r$. Similarly one dollar paid in two years' time would be worth one divided by $(1+r)^2$ today, while a dollar paid in 10 years' time would be worth one divided by $(1+r)^{10}$. This general process of expressing future payments in today's values is known as *discounting* while the rate used is often referred to as the *discount rate*. The further into the future a cost or a benefit occurs, the lower will be its value today.

These techniques are important for all activities where benefits or costs occur over a number of years. In this situation, values must be expressed in present terms so that they can be summed on an equal basis; it may also be useful to compare this project with other possible interventions, whose costs and benefits have a different distribution over time. (For simple examples of the use of discounting, see Creese & Parker, 1994, and the example used in section 8.7 of this book.)

3.3.4 Which discount factor should be used?

When doing economic appraisal, it is easiest if all costs and benefits are expressed in *real terms*—without inflating figures to include an allowance for inflation. The discount factor should, therefore, also be a real rate of discount. Arguably, uncertainty should also be disregarded since the government is the investor and is large enough to absorb the risk associated with projects (and besides, uncertainty is not cumulative and consistently negative, as the discount rate would imply). Many people also dispute the argument about diminishing marginal utility: first, because it may be wrong to assume that society will always get richer, and secondly because, if it does, the effect of increasing income levels may be offset by the fact that health is a luxury good (hence as you get richer, each unit of health is likely to have more value).

The choice of discount rates for health projects is therefore contentious. This is natural, since discount rates express *inter-temporal equity* (how much are the interests of future people worth, relative to our own?), and are therefore at root a political decision. However, there is a consensus that discount rates based on the *social rate of time preference* should be applied. The rate that is often used is the real return on a low risk asset such as government bonds. Thus, if the rate of return payable is 15% and the inflation rate is 10% then the discount rate that is used is 5%. There is also something to be said for using the same rate as in published studies. This is generally around 5 or 6%. This is particularly important in countries where the official nominal interest is very high while the real rate is negative as prices are rising very rapidly. Using a rate from published studies may come closer to a long-term world rate of discount.

3.3.4.1   Vaccination example: part 2

Let us assume that the vaccination programme (whether polyclinic- or community-based) is to continue indefinitely at the same rate of annual activity. In this case it is easiest to annualise the costs of the capital items rather than discount all costs to their present value. Assume that, for the building, its expected life is 20 years. Assume that the cold-storage compartment and vehicle have life expectancies of five years. The discount rate is 5%. The cost profile for the polyclinic and community-based outreach programme vaccination campaign is given in Table 3.3. The annualised capital costs are given in columns (3) and (5).

These are produced by obtaining the annual payment over the lifetime of the item that, when discounted, gives the original cost. It is higher than simply dividing the total cost by the number of years of use since it includes the interest foregone (opportunity cost) by investing in the capital item rather than putting the equivalent money into a bank account.

It is assumed that 300 vaccinations are given out each month under the community programme, 200 under the polyclinic-based scheme.

The cost per vaccination in this hypothetical programme is given as 1.72 for the polyclinic programme and 1.64 for the community programme. Although the capital costs of the community programme are higher, the higher level of activity, based on the assumption that more children will be reached by taking the programme to the community, enables the unit costs to be lower. It should be noted that this result is based on the assumption that any spare

Table 3.3   Costs of the polyclinic and community programme

	Polyclinic programme		Community programme	
	Total cost	Annual cost	Total cost	Annual cost
(1)	(2)	(3)	(4)	(5)
Capital				
Building	450	36.11		
Cold storage	2000	461.95	2000	461.95
Vehicle			5000	1154.87
Total capital		498.06		1616.82
Recurrent				
Staff		3000		4000
Vaccines		120		180
Other		500		100
Total recurrent		3620		4280
Total vaccinations (per year)		2400		3600
Recurrent + capital		4118.06		5896.82
Cost per vaccination		1.72		1.64

capacity in the polyclinic as a consequence of carrying out fewer vaccinations will be used for some other programme. If this is not the case, then the opportunity cost (i.e. the benefits foregone) of the building will be lower—a factor which could change the final result.

3.3.5   Sensitivity analysis

In any economic appraisal there will be uncertainty about some of the assumptions that are made. For example, the discount rate might be lower, the cost of a vehicle may change, or the number of vaccinations that can be carried out by the outreach team might be overestimated. Sometimes a change in an assumption will have little impact on the final result; sometimes the impact can be quite substantial, changing the conclusion completely. Any well-formulated economic appraisal will carry out a sensitivity analysis that *tests how sensitive a result is to changes in key parameters*. Parameters should be varied within expected limits since there is little point in testing the effect of a scenario that almost certainly will not occur. For example, if historical information suggests that the real rate of interest never fluctuates below 2% or above 10% then testing the effect of a 20% rate is probably unnecessary and misleading. In contrast, it would be desirable to test the effect of a range of rates betwen 2 and 10%.

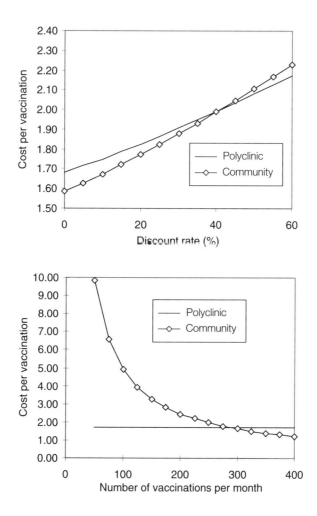

Figure 3.2   Sensitivity analysis using example data

3.3.5.1   Vaccination example: part 3

In Figure 3.2, the results are presented of sensitivity tests that vary the discount rate and number of vaccinations performed in the community using the hypothetical data. The results show that the rate of discount only changes the choice of community over hospital care when the real rate of interest reaches around 40%. Since this is very unlikely, this factor can probably be ignored. In contrast, varying the number of vaccinations performed in the uncertain setting of the outreach programme can have a major impact on the choice. A reduction of just 20 vaccinations per month is enough to make the polyclinic programme superior. This result suggests that further investigation on the probable number of vaccinations that can be carried out in each programme would be valuable in informing the final decision.

3.4   COST-EFFECTIVENESS ANALYSIS

Cost-minimisation analysis is a way of comparing the costs of two or more ways of achieving the same output or outcome. If, however, there are reasons to suppose that the outcome of the programmes are different, then more sophisticated analysis is required that allows alternative outcomes to be compared. Cost-effectiveness analysis (CEA) allows two projects to be compared that achieve the same objective but do so with different levels of success. Programmes could either be different ways of treating the same condition or treatment of different diseases that have the same major objective, such as reduction in deaths or days lost from work. The crucial requirement for CEA is that *benefits are expressed in some common unit*.

The most common units used are *life years gained* or *deaths averted*. Of these two, the first is the most precise since it examines the length of the life gained as a result of the treatment. However, it requires considerably more information on survival and complication rates. The second is useful if the prevention of a death is equivalent between programmes. For example, two successful but different vaccination programmes that prevent individuals contracting the same potentially fatal diseases can be assumed to lead to a similar extension of life.

To calculate deaths averted, three pieces of information are required if the intervention is curative in scope:

- number of cases treated;
- effectiveness of the treatment; and
- case fatality rates (CFR).

If the intervention is preventive, then the probability of contracting the disease should be added to the equation.

The product of these data determines the number of deaths averted.

$$\text{Cost per death prevented} = \frac{\text{Annual programme cost}}{\text{CFR} \times \text{efficacy} \times \text{number treated} \times \text{probability of contracting disease}}$$

For example, in the case of vaccinations illustrated above, if the efficacy of the vaccine is 85%, the case fatality rate is 5%, the probability of contracting the disease, if unvaccinated, is 5%, and the number of people vaccinated is 3600, then the number of deaths averted would be 7.65. Cost-effectiveness ratios can then be obtained by dividing the cost of the intervention by the number of deaths averted.

Computation of life years gained is a more relevant concept than deaths averted for comparison of most curative, particularly surgical, procedures. Knowledge of complications and mortality are required and may utilise either retrospective data from past studies, or carry out prospective cohort studies on patients undergoing treatment. A common period of follow-up for patients is 10 years. Prospective studies are more likely to give accurate results but take longer and cost more to implement. If there are reliable studies that have already demonstrated the effectiveness of the procedures, then these data may be adequate for computing benefits.

Cost-effectiveness analysis allows programmes that achieve similar benefits to be compared. Since ratios are derived the technique cannot say whether any of the programmes being compared are worth doing in absolute terms—there is no way of saying whether the procedure is rendering more in benefits than it is costing. It is also not possible to compare programmes that have different effects. For example, it would not be appropriate to use CEA to compare the effects of hip-replacement with intensive care for low birthweight babies; the first produces little extension to life but may enhance quality, while the foremost objective of the second is to prolong life. To do this other methods are required.

3.5   COST–BENEFIT ANALYSIS

Cost–benefit analysis (CBA) goes one stage further than CEA in expressing benefits as well as costs in monetary terms. By doing this, programmes with completely different effects can be compared. It is also possible to say whether a programme is making a net contribution to society by examining whether benefits exceed costs.

The central problem with this technique is that it is frequently very difficult to place a money value on many of the benefits being considered. This problem is perhaps most clearly seen in placing a *monetary value on human life*, which will be a benefit of many medical interventions. A number of different techniques have been used to do this. One method (the *human capital approach*) values life in terms of the discounted productive capacity of the patient treated. The implication of this approach, however, is that if an unemployed or a retired person is treated, the value of his or her life is worth less than a person that is working. Typically, unpaid workers such as housewives or subsistence farmers tend also to be undervalued under this approach.

A different approach is to try to get individuals to set a monetary value on life, health, mobility etc. This can be done by direct questioning (contingent valuation) or through indirect means, such as observation of their behaviour, or the behaviour of public officials. All of these methods raise a number of methodological issues.

3.5.1 Contingent valuation

This involves asking people what they would be prepared to pay to avoid a given condition or what they would consider to be acceptable compensation for having it. The question can be put in a definite form, or giving probabilities of different health states. In terms of the valuation, it can be open ended, or with a suggested scale of payments. The problems, however, are numerous:

- It is very open to bias according to who asks the questions, how they are asked etc. For example, studies generally get different results if the question is about treating a condition rather than preventing it.
- The respondent is open to suggestion, for example, where a payments scale is used.
- Who should be questioned? Patients? Potential patients? Their relatives? Doctors? Society at large? All will have different perspectives and values.
- The payments are likely to correlate with income levels, so a representative sample of income levels must be included.
- The information which the respondent requires can be very complex, specifying different options, probabilities, side-effects etc.
- It is not always clear what is being valued (is it pain relief? dignity? reassurance? mobility?).
- More basically, how do you set a monetary value on life? Are people able to trade-off such unlike goods?

Not surprisingly, then, studies using these methods to assess the value of one human life have come up with a very wide range of values, from 69 000 US$ to 10 million US$ (most studies were conducted in the US). Even if the methodology is refined, the results are likely to remain localised. It should also be noted that the values are private—i.e. do not incorporate any externalities, which must be accounted for separately.

3.5.2 Indirect methods

These methods focus on private or public behaviour and the values which these imply for a human life, or prevention of disability etc. For example, differentials in pay between jobs involving different measures of physical risk may be taken to be a proxy for the value which individuals set on life or health, or payments on life insurance as an indication of the value of that life. In the public arena, court awards may be taken to indicate the value attached by the public to a human life, or the amount set aside by the legislature for public safety measures to indicate the value placed by society on health. The problem is that these proxies are rarely very accurate.

Pay differentials, for example, reflect many considerations such as skills required, job satisfaction, labour mobility, degree of local unemployment, power of the local unions etc. Health hazards may play only a very minor part in the establishment of wages. Or, in the case of life insurance, the amount is likely to reflect whether the person taking it out is risk averse or a risk-taker, and, if the former, how much they think their family will need to live on in the event of their death. This is not the same as the intrinsic value which they set on their own life. As for public bodies, they will reflect very specific conditions, such as whether it is an election year when the law is passed, how strong the lobby group in favour of the measure is, etc. Moreover, it would be an example of circular reasoning to use the value implicit in the behaviour of public bodies to better inform the work of public bodies (most valuation exercises being carried out for that purpose).

While cost–benefit analysis appears to be a more flexible technique than cost-effectiveness analysis, the difficulty in valuing health benefits limits its operation in practice. Most studies that employ the approach, analyse interventions that provide clear financial benefits (such as increased productivity at work) but where reduction in death or discomfort is low.

3.6   COST–UTILITY ANALYSIS

The need to combine measures of quality and amount of life gained from different interventions together with difficulty in placing money valuations on these benefits has led to the development of *cost–utility analysis* (CUA).

One way of ranking diverse benefits of different health care interventions is to look at the value or utility society places upon different health states. There are a number of ways that are used to obtain such valuations, but most attempt to place health states on a scale from one (representing perfect health) through zero (representing death); negative values are permitted on the basis that there may be some states that individuals consider worse than death. Treatments can then be valued according to how much they increase this *health status index*, multiplied by years of life added. Those that mainly improve the quality of life can be compared to those that mainly increase the quantity of life.

Individual valuation of health states can be obtained through interviews and questionnaires. A number of indexes have been developed, including the quality-adjusted life year (*QALY*, or its offspring, the *EuroQual*), years of healthy life (*YHE*) and the disability adjusted life year (*DALY*). By utilising cost data, the cost of obtaining one quality-adjusted year can be calculated for a range of treatments. Choices in purchasing might, in theory, be based on such calculations with money being spent first on treatments that offer the lowest cost health gain, then the second lowest continuing down the list until resources are used up. For an early example of this approach, see Williams (1985). Analysis of this kind is, however, still in its infancy and there are many problems of methodology and application still to be resolved. A full critique is provided in Carr-Hill (1989).

Some district health authorities in the UK are already beginning to use QALY-type tables to rank health care interventions in order to inform priority setting. The World Bank *World Development Report* of 1993 uses DALYs to compare the burden of disease across countries and regions (including the former Soviet bloc) and as a tool for prioritising between different interventions in terms of cost effectiveness. Purchasers should be cautious about the use of league tables, however; in particular, the basis on which costs and benefits are calculated should be the same for each activity, samples should be adequate, and the parameters used (e.g. discount rates, preference rankings) should be locally applicable.

3.7   CONCLUSION

Decisions in the health sector of different levels of complexity can be informed by the use of economic analysis. At its most simple, techniques have been developed to compare the costs of two interventions to determine which is the cheapest, assuming that they both achieve the same results. At its most complicated, economic analysis tries to compare activities which achieve

---

Box 3.3   Principles of economic evaluation (Coyle & Davies: Reproduced with permission from Drummond & Maynard (eds) *Purchasing and providing cost effective health care* © 1993 Churchill Livingstone)

1. The study question perspective and design should be clearly stated.
2. The study should involve a comparison of at least two alternatives. The 'do nothing', least costly and most-used options should be considered.
3. All relevant costs and benefits of the alternatives should be identified and appropriately valued.
4. The study should be of a sufficient size to assess significant differences between alternatives.
5. The marginal costs and benefits of alternatives should be valued.
6. Future costs and benefits should be appropriately discounted.
7. Detailed sensitivity analysis should be conducted.

different results for different groups of people, which involves methods for quantifying values and feelings, if not in money, then at least on some scale which can be aggregated. Despite the difficulties, economists persist in trying new ways of doing this, because the alternative to maximising gain is a purely political or random approach to allocating resources between different activities.

Further discussion of economic evaluation and its uses will be found in the following chapter on purchasing.

REFERENCES AND FURTHER READING

Carr-Hill, R. (1989) Assumptions of the QALY process. *Social Science and Medicine*, vol. 29, no. 3, pp. 469–477.

Coyle, D. & Davies, L. (1993) How to assess cost-effectiveness: elements of a sound economic evaluation, in Drummond & Maynard, op. cit.

Creese, A. & Parker, D., eds (1994) *Cost analysis in primary health care: a training manual for programme managers*. Geneva: World Health Organisation (basic but practical guide to costing issues).

Drummond, M. & Maynard, A., eds (1993) *Purchasing and providing cost-effective health care*. London: Churchill Livingstone.

Drummond, M., Stoddart, G. & Torrance, G. (1987) *Methods for the economic evaluation of health care programmes*. Oxford: Oxford University Press.

Sheldon, T., Song, F. & Davey Smith, G. (1993) Critical appraisal of the medical literature, in Drummond & Maynard, op. cit.

Stevens, A. & Raftery, J., eds (1994) *Health care needs assessment*, vols 1 and 2. Oxford: Radcliffe Medical Press.

Williams, A. (1985) Economics of coronary artery bypass grafting. *British Medical Journal*, vol. 291, pp. 326–329.

World Development Report 1993: Investing in health. Washington, DC: World Bank.

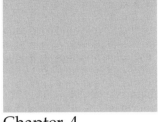

Chapter 4

PURCHASING HEALTH CARE

Sophie Witter

4.1 INTRODUCTION

As discussed in Chapter 1, patients find themselves in an *agency relationship* with doctors because of the asymmetry of information about diagnosis and different methods of potential treatment. They are therefore in a weak position to bargain with doctors, who also represent their own interests as providers of health care. It is important then to have bodies which represent patient interests and the public interest (as funders of health care and because of the externalities associated with health problems) in negotiating with providers. These are known as 'purchasers'.

Until recently, in many countries the function of assessing health needs at a population level and buying services to meet those needs was integrated with the organisation of the provision of health services. However, problems of technical inefficiency (such as lack of incentives for staff to work hard) and allocative inefficiency (such as supply-led services) were common. Current reorganisations are therefore tending to stress a 'market model' in which buyers are represented by health purchasers (such as health authorities or insurance companies) and sellers are represented by providers (such as family practitioners or hospitals). This development has been known in the UK as the *purchaser–provider split*.

This chapter will focus on the role of health purchaser. What should they do, and how can their position be strengthened? This last question arises from the weak position in which purchasers often find themselves, both in the former Soviet bloc and elsewhere. Even though they have the financial muscle (from public finances or insurance contributions), purchasers are often dominated by the interests of professionals within the provider agencies or follow historic funding patterns without reviewing the cost effectiveness and appropriateness of the services being provided. Where insurers are mainly

An Introduction to Health Economics for Eastern Europe and the Former Soviet Union.
Edited by Sophie Witter and Tim Ensor. © 1997 John Wiley & Sons, Ltd.

concerned with attracting customers (e.g. in a private voluntary insurance system), it can be particularly difficult to plan services. The importance of this *'thinking role'* within the health service requires fresh emphasis.

The issue of how the purchaser's budget is set will not be discussed in detail. When finance is raised through public taxation or social insurance, the most common approach is to allocate budgets by geographical area on the basis of a *weighted capitation formula*. The weightings may be based on estimates of need, such as deviations from standardised mortality rates for the country; variations in service delivery cost; and indicators of social deprivation, such as unemployment rates. For further details, see Bevan (1989).

4.2 DIFFERENT TYPES OF PURCHASERS

The overall objective of a purchaser is usually to maximise improvements in the health status of the population in the area concerned, and this is done through needs assessment and the purchasing of effective and cost-effective services (see Table 4.1). Lower level objectives may include such criteria for services as accessibility, quality, appropriateness etc.

Essentially, purchasers are allocating resources for a given area or population within the health service—providing limits within which doctors can allocate resources between individual patients, according to their clinical judgement. The way in which they do this will depend on the structure of the health market.

In purely private systems, resources will be allocated according to the financial status and perceived health needs of the individual, leaving little role for population-based purchasing.

In an insurance market which is concerned with cost escalation, a number of options for controlling resource allocation exist. One is to try to improve technical efficiency of services through price controls and/or clinical protocols, using instruments like *DRGs* (*diagnostic-related groups*, discussed further under payments for providers). These aim to limit the costs per medical intervention, but do not affect the numbers treated or the pattern of services itself. Another approach is through *'managed care'*, which sets fixed budgets for health care per patient per year, thus providing incentives to limit unnecessary care (see Chapter 5 for details). This system does provide some incentives for allocative efficiency, but only within the relatively small population seen by each particular provider group.

Where a purchaser has a relatively stable income and operates on behalf of a large, known population, it has the option of *planning services on a population*

Table 4.1 Stages in purchasing: purchasing roles and activities

1. Assess needs of population.
2. Examine cost-effective strategies to meet needs (including preventive strategies).
3. Relate to existing services to identify room for positive change (in quantity or quality).
4. Consult public/patients/doctors on social values and priorities.
5. Draw up health care objectives and priorities.
6. Based on these, draw up contract specifications.
7. Sign contracts with providers, agreeing on quantity, quality and cost of services.
8. Monitor performance of providers, directly and by taking views of public/doctors etc.
9. Feedback this information into next round of needs assessment, priority setting and contracting.

basis. This is the model which this chapter will concentrate on, although the activities described here will also apply to other purchasers to varying degrees, depending on their scope for allocating resources. Even if patients have free choice between provider agencies, the purchasers in most countries still play an important role in planning of new investments and infrastructure development of providers.

The role of *market regulator* is one which should in theory be distinct from that of purchaser, though in many countries they are combined or overlap (particularly where there is only one purchaser for an area). A market regulator deals with such issues as entry and exit rules, making provision for market stability, quality control, rules of competition, and licensing of agents (see Arvidsson, 1995, for further discussion of market regulation). This is a role which is best played by a national-level body.

4.3   NEEDS ASSESSMENT

4.3.1   Definitions and perspectives

The concept of need is highly ambiguous. What you think you need and what I think you need are very likely to be different: in other words, it depends on who is doing the judging. A common distinction is therefore made by health economists between:

- *wants*, which refer to the subjective desires of a person, reflecting their personal characteristics as well as the information available to them;
- *objective needs*, which refers to their 'real' health care requirements (if we could know them);

- *normative needs*, which reflect an expert's judgement about what is needed, which in turn reflects changing medical knowledge and fashions, among other things;
- *demands*, which are wants made concrete through an action, such as purchasing a service (i.e. requiring not only a desire but also the decision and ability to act on that desire, such as having enough money to do so, if services are not free); and
- *capacity to benefit*, which unites the concept of objective need with the availability of effective treatments to meet that need.

All these are distinct again from *priorities*, which can be defined as the public decision-makers understanding of needs, filtered through a net of political considerations.

Health economists are concerned with maximising health gains ('adding years to life and life to years') and therefore tend to use the definition relating to capacity to benefit. They, like purchasers (and indeed public health specialists), take a *community-wide perspective*, which can conflict with the doctor's approach, which is to provide the best treatment available for the individual patient whom he or she is treating. The problem with the individual approach is that it does not take account of the people who do not present themselves to the doctor; it also typically fails to take account of the cost of treatments (and thus of its *opportunity costs*: the treatments which other people forego as a result).

The argument for having an explicit goal like maximising health gains is that it forces doctors, managers and politicians to be clear about their priorities. The alternative in health care (where the demand is ever growing but the resources are fixed) is to have *rationing based on less explicit principles*, such as provider preference, or patronage links, or first-come-first-served.

The principle of maximising health gains has an implicit assumption that one unit of health gain (say, one year of life gained, adjusted for quality) will have an equal value, regardless of who is gaining it. However, this can be modified to reflect social values: if, for example, there is a consensus that health gains are more valuable for young people, then these can be weighted to reflect that feeling. Purchasers therefore have the task not only of assessing capacity to benefit in an objective way, but also of *incorporating social values* in their decisions.

4.3.2   How needs are determined

If needs are interpreted as capacity to benefit, then three types of information are required to determine them:

- *epidemiological*: the prevalence and incidence of disease in the population;
- *medical/economic*: the effectiveness and cost effectiveness of treatments available for these diseases (see previous chapter); and
- *institutional*: the services which currently exist to meet those needs.

An analysis of all three areas should produce insights into how service patterns should be changed to maximise health gains, either by expanding or cutting back services.

Relevant epidemiological information includes the size and age structure of the population, standardised mortality rates, and data on the incidence and prevalence of diseases in the population. These are usually obtained from general censuses, hospital epidemiological records and national prevalence studies. They are analysed by public health specialists and compared with other areas of roughly similar population composition in order to spot areas of underachievement or *comparative need*. Data published by the Ministry of Health presenting comparisons of health indicators nationally can assist local purchasers in their task.

However, disease patterns alone cannot dictate services, as many if not most of the factors producing good or bad health lie outside the control of the health sector (such as income distribution, nutrition, education, physical environment, social attitudes etc.). It is therefore important to identify the problems which can be *addressed effectively within the health sector* and prioritise them according to resource availability.

Purchasers need access to information about medical effectiveness and cost effectiveness (see last chapter), and also need to interpret how far that information is accurate and relevant to their local situation. Preferences and costs in particular are likely to vary from place to place. The acceptability of a service, which directly influences effectiveness, will also vary according to cultural and socio-economic factors.

Finally, purchasers need to ascertain to what extent current services are meeting the needs which have been identified, using effective interventions. The issue here is not merely whether services exist, but also whether they are of an *adequate quality* and are being *utilised*. This can be judged technically, using clinical audits, but also from the point of view of patients, using vehicles like patient satisfaction surveys.

4.4 WIDER CONSULTATION

In Table 4.1 a process of wider consultation is neatly placed between needs assessment and drawing up health care objectives and priorities. In reality, though, consultation is on-going and will occur at all stages of the planning cycle. There are a number of reasons for encouraging consultation:

- to ascertain *demand* and social weightings for potential health gains (to influence cost-effectiveness calculations);
- to build up *local and national support* for health services (political consideration);
- to ensure that different interest groups are treated fairly (*equity*); and
- to inform *rationing decisions*, where it is accepted that public finances will not meet the full range of health needs of a population.

There are three main groups with whom purchasers will usually seek to consult: community representatives, professionals and national government.

4.4.1 Community representatives

Purchasers usually live locally and are therefore likely to be influenced by expressions of concern, whether these take the form of media pressure, actions by local politicians or complaints by the general public. Typically, these put an upward pressure on demand for services and make it particularly hard to change existing service patterns.

More formally, a system of *community councils* can be established to liaise between the general public and purchasers. Members could be elected to these, or co-opted by existing members, or hold office on the basis of their other positions. Commonly, however, such bodies suffer from a lack of authority, both because their representativeness is open to question (especially when unelected) and because they have little power to influence decisions, relative to doctors, managers and politicians. Even if purchasers are motivated to listen to consumers, it can be hard to reconcile what is wanted with what can be afforded, and to reconcile professional and non-professional perceptions.

Where contacts with the community are often most constructive is in *investigating specific issues*, such as why there is a low utilisation of services among a particular group, or what type of service is preferred by specific client groups. Acting on such inputs is easiest when the findings accord with cost-effectiveness information (e.g. transfer of treatments from hospitals to primary care settings) or where the cost implications of changes are at least neutral.

Recently there have been some experiments aiming to involve more meaningfully representatives of the local community in setting priorities for health services. In Oregon State, USA, this was done by getting representatives of the public to prioritise between services to be provided on Medicare/Medicaid (i.e. paid for by public funding). These value judgements were then combined with consideration of cost and health gain to produce a ranking of interventions, which could be tailored to the resources available to buy them. Such a process is sophisticated and time-consuming, and may not be suitable for all types of treatments (in Oregon, mental health, substance abuse and drug addiction were excluded).

4.4.2 Professionals

Consultation with professionals will take varying forms, such as informal discussions with individuals, or regular meetings with bodies representing general practitioners (GPs), for example, or social services organisations, and meetings with trade unions to discuss issues of concern to staff.

4.4.3 National government

Purchasers also have to try to meet with national policies, which may be expressed in terms of essential services or target outcomes. For example, in the UK the Department of Health published a document entitled 'Health of the nation', which set for the first time specific national targets for reductions in mortality in five areas (see Department of Health, 1992). In this case, the areas were heart disease and strokes, cancer, accidents, AIDS and sexual health, and mental health. More recently, other target areas such as environmental health have been added. At the minimum this is a statement of political prioritisation. More optimistically, it may encourage health managers to take a broader look at the factors behind ill-health and form alliances across bureaucratic boundaries to address them.

The degree of responsiveness to government policies will depend ultimately on financial levers: for example, it might be easier to achieve in an integrated system, than in one where insurers are paid directly by households or firms.

4.5 PRIORITISING AND SETTING OBJECTIVES

Purchasers' planning tools can take different forms, depending on the time horizon which is adopted.

- Ideally, *objectives* should be set first, either in terms of improved health status or reduction of burden of specific diseases. These would be expected to take some years to achieve, depending on the objectives themselves.
- A *strategy* can then be outlined which states the changes in services which are needed to achieve the objectives.
- This, in turn, can inform the detailed *annual plans* of what to buy, from whom, and at what price.

This process also provides a framework for *monitoring*, which should relate both to activities (services: quality, cost and quantity) and outcomes (changes in health status).

Economists often assume a *zero-based approach* in which all current investment has to be thoroughly reviewed and justified. However, in most cases, the bulk of current activities are accepted as given, with purchasers looking for *gains at the margin*. Armed with information about 'good buys' in health care and the opinions of the public (however constituted), purchasers can identify areas for expansion or reduction of services. For example, they might decide to increase the allocation of resources to primary care, microsurgery and joint replacements and to decrease funding for services considered less effective, such as tonsillectomies, or less essential, such as cosmetic forms of plastic surgery.

Comparative analysis is also powerful. If utilisation rates for a particular service are low, relative to other areas, purchasers might either identify the reasons for this low level (where the service is considered to be important) and seek to address these OR negotiate a reduction in the level and/or cost of service provided. Differential costs between regions and differential rates of intervention for the same condition are also signals which would prompt further investigation by purchasers.

Valid strategies include not only the increase or decrease of a service as such, but also shifts within a service, for example, from treatment to prevention; changes in which facility provides the service (e.g. secondary to primary care shift); and also managerial changes such as improved co-ordination of services for a client group such as the mentally ill. It may also relate to activities carried out by the purchasers themselves—for example, public health measures or health education, where these are carried out by purchasing agencies.

The main constraint is *resource availability*, and because purchasers have to keep within fixed financial limits for the year they may have to make trade-offs—for example, between the quantity of services provided and their quality, or between different health objectives which can be pursued. There may also be conflicts between decisions based on effectiveness and *political and equity considerations* (e.g. if one client group loses out to another, or one geographical area to another, or even one group of doctors to another). There is no formula for resolving these and in practice some sort of pragmatic compromise may be necessary.

4.6 RELATIONSHIPS WITH PROVIDERS

Contracting and monitoring performance will be discussed in detail in the sections dealing with health providers. However, we must note here the

---

Box 4.1 The Wakefield prioritisation process (Adapted from Watson, Horne & Firth, 1996)

It is much harder to disinvest in existing activities than it is to assess the value of taking on new commitments. Wakefield Health Authority in the UK used a process to assess proposals for new activities, which provides an interesting example of one way of carrying out this type of selection.

The health authority first invited proposals for funding for the following financial year (1995–96). These were then marked according to a number of criteria:

1. *Potential health gain.* A panel of experts was asked to grade each intervention according to the degree of expected benefit (from 'life saving with full recovery', 6 points, through to 'improvement in service quality with no direct effect on fatality, disability or pain', 1 point). These points were added to points for numbers of people affected, ranging from 1 for 'up to 10' to 6 for 'over 10 000'. The maximum score for health gain was thus 12, which made up 24% of the maximum overall potential score of 50.
2. *Strength of evidence of clinical effectiveness.* The panel also gave scores for the strength of the evidence used to support the effectiveness of the intervention, ranging from 9 for 'several RCTs or of unchallengeable benefit' to 0 for 'no controlled studies'.
3. *Favouring prevention.* As this was a criteria for the health authority, activities preventing disease were given additional marks in comparison with curative interventions for that same condition. The highest mark here was 9 for 'intervention prevents a problem for which there is no specific treatment' to 3 for 'intervention prevents a problem where total relief is possible'.
4. *Appropriate setting.* Activities which took place in a setting which improved patient access were given additional marks, assuming that clinical effectiveness was maintained. The score was 6 for more appropriate setting, 4 for no change, and 2 for less appropriate setting.
5. *Promotion of equity.* Developments which promoted equity within the Wakefield district (either in terms of geographical inequality or by providing services to groups with particular problems) were awarded 6 marks; those which were thought to bring the district more into line with other districts were awarded 4 marks; and those which might make an existing service more acceptable to its target population were awarded 2 points.
6. *Public preference.* A panel of members of the public were asked to list their top five services in order of preference, with bids grouped into broad service areas. The top five were then given scores of 0 to 4, which amounted to 8% of the total score of 50.
7. *GP preference.* Each practice in the district was written to, asking them to list their top five preferences out of 35 bids. These votes were then used to give scores of 0 to 4, as for the public preference, thus giving GPs an influence over 8% of the total marks.

Discussion

The Wakefield process is interesting as it uses a set of explicit criteria, each of which is given a specific weight within the decision-making process. Bids are then graded according to these, by the general public and doctors as well as managers and public health specialists, and given a final ranking.

A number of criticisms can be made of the method. For example, there is no consideration of cost during the gradings. You could also argue that the number of people expected to be affected should be multiplied by expected health gains, not summed. The weights given to different considerations and different groups is also necessarily arbitrary.

More importantly, though, the process assumes that development funds will be available, but in many health services these funds are simply not available, as resources are fully consumed by on-going activities which are excluded from review. This severely limits the usefulness of this process, which is of course time-consuming and expensive in itself.

importance of the nature of the relationship between purchaser and providers and the *degree of competition* which prevails in the provider market.

Where, for example, there is only one major hospital in the area and strong historic links between that hospital and the health authority, it will be difficult to achieve gains from competition with the introduction of quasi-market or internal market systems. With the provider in a *monopolistic position*, it may well increase its prices and thus decrease social welfare.

Alternatively, where there are a number of providers, the purchaser may have to contemplate allowing the weaker ones to lose business and ultimately cease to operate. Given the historical relationship between them and the attachment of local people to local hospital facilities, this can be very politically contentious. This has been the case in London, in the UK, where inner city hospitals have faced closure or the need to merge with other facilities to survive.

The balancing act is for purchasers to *encourage the long-term health of providers* so as to ensure a degree of competition and also stability in the market, while *not colluding with provider interests* at the expense of patients and the public interest.

A further issue is the *transfer of information* about the processes and costs of production of health care: purchasers will seek this because they want to get the 'biggest bang for their buck' and also have an interest in the long-term survival and efficiency of providers; providers, however, no longer have to or want to divulge what is commercially sensitive information. In the absence of a competitive environment, this secrecy can make it very difficult for purchasers to negotiate reductions in prices or gains in quality.

4.7   COMPETITION BETWEEN PURCHASERS

It may be the case that a single purchaser exists, with responsibility for a whole population (i.e. *monopsony*, or a single buyer), and that competitive forces are restricted to the realm of providers. However, it is also common to find competition between purchasers, either in the same area or between areas. Private insurance companies, for example, or Health Maintenance Organisations in the US, operate as competing purchasers within an area. In theory this provides an incentive for them to increase their own efficiency, although in practice it is not easy to judge purchaser performance.

The same constraint applies in a public system where competition takes the form of a central government agency such as the Ministry of Health monitoring the performance of purchasers in different regions and setting targets and guidelines for them (i.e. a more regulatory approach). Some measure of *purchaser 'value added'* is required, which takes into account the original health state of the population and the strengths and weaknesses of local providers. On the basis of that information, we could in theory calculate how much health gain has been 'produced' by purchaser policies, and reward them accordingly. Clearly this calls for a highly sophisticated information system, which might in itself not be cost effective, especially if there are no financial incentives to reward high-performing purchasers or punish poor ones.

Within a publically funded and free system it is possible to have competition between purchasers within the same area, such as has occurred in the UK since the introduction of *GP fundholding*. A portion or all of the budget per capita for referral services is now held by general practitioners (GPs) who have opted to be fundholding, who purchase services for their patients directly from the referral centres. This may have the effect of giving higher priority to patient interests (although it is debatable to what extent these benefits accrue to the whole population rather than creating a two-tier system with priority given to patients of fundholding GPs). In such situations, it would make sense for *purchasers to co-ordinate their policies* so as to give coherent signals to providers, or else to specialise in different functions (e.g. budgets devolved to GPs, with health authorities setting the strategic framework, providing health intelligence, and supporting GPs in comparing performance and improving the quality of services bought).

As with providers, it may also be the case that there are *economies of scale or scope for purchasers*—i.e. a reduction in average costs as numbers increase or as range of functions increase—such that the gains from efficiency would be more than offset by increased costs. This would be an argument in favour of larger purchasing agencies, in terms of area covered: they should be able to make better use of information systems, staff and equipment, as well as having increased bargaining power in relation to providers.

A different option for providing competition between purchasers would be a *managed market* system under which patients choose between competing insurers or funding bodies, which are paid risk-related premia from a central fund (based on income-related contributions) and which in turn set up contracts with primary and secondary providers. This system was the basis for the Clinton proposals in the United States and the Dekker proposals in the Netherlands, and is beginning to be practised in certain regions of Russia (see Sheiman, 1994).

This might be regarded as an optimal arrangement in terms of maximising competitive forces within the system. However, the usual information problems arise: if it is hard for the Ministry of Health to judge purchaser performance, how much more so for individuals choosing between purchasing agencies? We can also speculate that it might result in non-price competition and a shift towards attractive rather than essential services, as well as possibly increases in transaction costs for purchasers (see Robinson &

Luft, 1985, for evidence of non-price competition in the US). Significant amounts of resources are likely to be used on the development of the insurance companies (including some reserves or protection against their collpase) rather than being spent directly on patient care.

4.8   CONCLUSION

Purchasers of health care play a very important and complex role, which is more akin to an art than a science in most countries at present. In order to carry out their tasks effectively, they also need skilled personnel and computing systems which are sadly lacking in the former Soviet bloc at present.

In order to achieve *allocative efficiency* in the mix of services purchased, they require an ambitious range of information relating to:

- the effectiveness of interventions, in theory;
- their costs;
- the quantity required (which also influences costs); and
- their impact on health status in practice.

None of this is simple. Information on effectiveness is often scarce, or inaccessible, or even contradictory. Costs are hard to compare, given quality and other variations. Needs assessment is a complicated blend of elements; it cannot be assessed directly as if it were like the demand for food. Impact on health status is also very complicated in terms of establishing causal links.

Apart from problems of information, purchasers of health care also face *political, social and institutional pressures* and financial constraints. Thus, while the planning process should be informed by the rational model laid out in Table 4.1, there will invariably be guesses made and compromises sought.

In general, users of health care, protected in direct terms from costs, share with providers the desire to see health services increase in quantity. Hence the significance of the purchaser role, which is to *try to bring supply and demand more in line with need, defined as capacity to benefit*. This involves not only influencing supply via contracting, monitoring etc., but also influencing demand by activities like health promotion and education on the negative side-effects of drugs, for example.

This role of *'rationing'* health care is controversial, though. If people feel that they have a right to health care to meet all of their wants, then they are unlikely to accept the *utilitarian approach* taken by most health economists, which focuses not on individual rights but the widest benefit for the greatest number in society. In the USA, for example, this type of individualistic culture can be seen; it has its advantages in terms of standards of care for those who can afford it, but also major disadvantages in terms of cost escalation, patterns of service provided and access for those with lower incomes. (See Maxwell, 1995, for discussion of rationing issues.)

There is also a tension between the *advantages of size* in planning services and the *attractions of being 'close to' patients*. Thus in some systems, purchasing is effectively carried out by general practitioners or 'health maintenance organisations', which are chosen by patients and are thought to be more responsive to their needs. Planning for a whole district or area, on the other hand, offers economies of scale and scope and the potential to maximise overall health gain. This 'top-down' planning model is somewhat out of fashion at present, given the enthusiasm for market-based systems and consumer choice; however, it continues to offer certain advantages. In the UK and elsewhere, the government appears to be trying both approaches simultaneously, perhaps to allow the 'survival of the fittest'!

In many parts of the former Soviet bloc, it will take time for health authorities and insurance funds to evolve from a focus on maintaining a given medical infrastructure to being the agent of the insured and trying to maximise the value gained from resources invested in health. The first stage in this process may be to ensure that treatments are being provided in as efficient a manner as possible, by reviewing payments systems (see Chapter 5) and supporting the development of active management within provider agencies (see Chapter 6). The second stage might be to encourage effective treatment practice, for example by scrutinising variations between doctors or institutions, or, more proactively, by developing 'best practice' treatment protocols for specific diseases, involving both patients and doctors, and getting these into use. Finally, the issue of allocative efficiency and the distribution of resources between different activities must be addressed, through research on cost effectiveness locally and by tapping into international information networks (see Box 3.2).

REFERENCES AND FURTHER READING

Akehurst, R. & Ferguson, B. (1993) The purchasing authority, in Drummond, M. & Maynard, A., eds. *Purchasing and providing cost-effective health care*. London: Churchill Livingstone.
Arvidsson, G. (1995) Regulation of planned markets in health care, in Saltman, R. & Van Otter, C., eds, *Implementing planned markets in health care*. Buckingham: Open University Press.
Bevan, G. (1989) Financing UK hospital and community health services. *Oxford Review of Economic Policy*, vol. 5, no. 1. Oxford: Oxford University Press.
Department of Health (1992) *The health of the nation: a strategy for health in England*. London: HMSO.
Maxwell, R.J., ed. (1995) Rationing health care. *British Medical Journal*, vol. 51, no. 4, pp. 761–962.
Ovretveit, J. (1995) *Purchasing for health*. Buckingham: Open University Press.

Robinson, J. & Luft, H. (1985) The impact of hospital market structure on patient volume, average length of stay and costs of care. *Journal of Health Economics*, vol. 4, no. 4, pp. 333–357.

Sheiman, I. (1994) The development of market approaches in Russia. *International Journal of Health Planning and Management*, vol. 9, pp. 39–56.

Stevens, A. & Raftery, J. (1994) *Health care needs assessment.* Oxford: Radcliffe Medical Press.

Watson, P., Horne, G. & Firth, A. (1996) Assessing services: knowing the score. *Health Service Journal*, 14 March 1996, pp. 28–31.

Part IV

PROVIDING HEALTH SERVICES

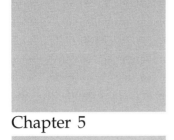

Chapter 5

METHODS OF PAYMENT TO MEDICAL CARE PROVIDERS

Tim Ensor, Sophie Witter and Igor Sheiman

An important theme in health economics is to separate consideration of the source of funding from the way in which resources are disbursed. These two issues are often confused, perhaps because certain payment systems are often associated with a given system for obtaining money. For example, fee for service payment is frequently linked with insurance-based systems, while salary and budget methods are linked with tax-funded systems. While this may often be the case, it need not be so: it is possible to have an insurance system that uses budgets to pay providers—as in Germany for hospitals—or a tax-funded system that makes use of fee for service payments.

This chapter will consider the main systems of provider payment and the *incentives* which they typically provide, in terms of service patterns, volume, quality and cost. The first part deals with payments for individual practitioners and the next with institutions, like hospitals. The focus in the first section is on payment for doctors' services, given their pivotal role in diagnosis, referral and treatment. In many contexts, however, the discussion applies equally as well to other health care staff such as nurses, dentists and paramedics, particularly where they exercise some autonomy in their clinical practice.

In its conclusion, the chapter will evaluate each method using the following criteria:

- cost of management and monitoring;
- ability to maintain overall cost containment;
- impact on technical efficiency; and
- quality of care.

An Introduction to Health Economics for Eastern Europe and the Former Soviet Union.
Edited by Sophie Witter and Tim Ensor. © 1997 John Wiley & Sons, Ltd.

Administrative cost and ease of monitoring is the cost of establishing the system and on-going cost of making payments and ensuring that the terms of the contract are met. Ability to maintain *cost containment* is the extent to which the payment system allows control over expenditure and prevents unnecessary treatment being provided. *Technical efficiency* is defined as the incentives that encourage providers to use resources in the most effective way to provide a particular service. (What type of service is provided will in turn depend on the demands of purchasers, which is a separate issue.) The final criterion is the way in which the system encourages providers to give a *good quality service* to patients.

5.1 PAYMENT OF MEDICAL STAFF

5.1.1 Salary

Using this system, the doctor is paid a fixed annual salary regardless of the quantity of work done and, frequently, the quality of treatment. This is the system predominant in most countries in transition where a medical practitioner has traditionally received a salary for life (usually at a level below the average wage). Income differentials between grades of staff were small and opportunities for material advancement were therefore few. The Soviet system did provide certain non-monetary rewards such as medals, study tours to other countries and accommodation. With the abolition of communism, though, many of these rewards have disappeared but nothing has been put in their place. Doctors must get by on declining real salaries combined with whatever extra they can earn from under-the-table payments or unofficial private work.

It is not surprising that the circumstances that doctors are currently faced with should lead many to want to replace salary payments with forms of fee for service payment. This is exacerbated by the observation that medical staff working in countries that make use of a fee system earn salaries that are often many times the average wage.

Although the desire to change the system is natural, it may be misplaced. Although salary payment may mean a job for life with no advancement, this need not be so. Salaried job contracts may be awarded for a limited term renewed on the basis of *meaningful performance review*. For example:

- various performance criteria may be included that allow for a modest increase in salary if certain levels of achievement are met;
- criteria may be included that allow for extra payments if certain targets (e.g. proportion vaccinated) are met;

- an employee may be offered fringe benefits such as research or travel opportunities (these were common under the Soviet regime as reward for compliance but they may also be offered for excellence); and
- other incentives include additional vacation and transport concessions.

The matter of who is selected to carry out *monitoring of performance* is very important. If it is a peer group, such as a group of senior doctors, then an emphasis may be placed on professional standards, but management objectives, to enable a hospital to meet a specific contract, may be ignored. In addition, they may be more willing to offer increments to all that apply, if they do not bear the financial consequences of their decision. In contrast, management-driven review may not concentrate enough upon professional or quality aspects of performance.

An equally and perhaps more important issue is the *level of payment* paid to workers. If a doctor can double his or her wage from informal payments, small increments from meeting performance targets are unlikely to be attractive. Although capitation (see section 5.1.3) has probably encouraged doctors to compete for a smaller number of patients in the UK, what was more important in persuading better doctors to become GPs was the increase in overall levels of remuneration (target income). This may also prove true in transition economies.

A number of policy options are available to allow this to happen, including retiring older doctors, putting some on to part-time contracts and regrading some as assistant doctors. Although none are popular, it is important that action is taken to prevent the best doctors leaving for higher salaries in the private sector.

5.1.2 Fee for service (FFS)

The fee for service method is dominant in continental Western European countries, the USA, Canada and Japan, for payment to both GPs and specialists. A specific amount is provided for each service. The physician itemises his or her services on a bill and the sickness fund pays the physician or reimburses the patient. This is the usual form of billing by self-employed physicians, both for ambulatory and hospital in-patient care.

The usual approach is that the medical association and the sickness funds negotiate the *fee schedule*, with the government providing guidelines to limit costs. A fee schedule is a relative-value scale giving each procedure a weight. A basic financial unit—*conversion factor*—is valued in money terms. To establish the cash payment to a doctor, it must be multiplied by the weight. The fee schedule stays essentially stable, but the conversion factor is usually increased each year or on a more regular basis if the rate of inflation is high.

The medical association receives from the payers the negotiated sum and reimburses the services of its members according to the number of units gained by each of them.

This payment system reflects the work actually done. The doctor has incentives to make the services he or she provides acceptable by attractive premises, prompt service and courtesy. The doctor is prepared to consult on matters which he or she may regard as trivial. Such doctors are interested to render as many services as possible. The weakness of the FFS method is that it encourages doctors to provide *more consultations and more expensive procedures*, some of which are not appropriate. A patient has to make repeat visits during the course of illness. Visit rates in countries using the FFS method are often more than twice as high as in countries with the capitation method. Such countries also have a relatively higher rate of prescribing drugs and diagnostic tests (Braham *et al.*, 1990). The emphasis tends to be on treatment, rather than prevention. If a doctor purchases a particular piece of equipment, there are strong financial incentives to use it frequently so as to pay off the capital cost as fast as possible. This has been a special problem for many continental Western European countries. Research has also found that twice as many operations are performed in countries where surgeons are paid according to their activity, rather than by salary (d'Intignano, 1992).

To compensate for this problem, the payer has to monitor claims closely and review doctors' performances. For example, in Germany sickness funds work out *'doctor profiles'* to reveal high-claim rates in particular services. Deviations from average figures show the pattern for each doctor. These profiles are circulated to doctors to expose the zones of excessive billing and to persuade high-claiming doctors to modify their performance. The payer may also insist on changes in the fee schedule to discourage provision of certain services. Some countries have issued formal requirements of *prior approvals* of the payer for the most expensive procedures.

Another method of cost control is used in Germany, where points are awarded to each procedure, but the *overall budget is fixed*, so that on the one hand the doctor has an incentive to be active, but ultimately, as a group, price is inversely related to volume, which allows expenditure ceilings to be set.

Although the weaknesses of the FFS method can partly be compensated by control mechanisms and also by introducing limits on expenditures, it remains cost-provoking and difficult to operate. It is not recommended for the countries of the former Soviet bloc for three main reasons:

1. Financial resources for health care are much more limited than in the Western countries. The inelastic supply of resources to the system makes the ability to *ration* health care more important.

2. The FFS method does not encourage *preventive activity*. The great under-
    funding of the health sector in the former Soviet bloc, as well as the
    lifestyle-related burden of disease, makes preventive work by physicians a
    priority, as well as being more cost effective.
3. *Cost sharing* as a tool against overbilling is not acceptable in countries like
    Russia for political reasons.

5.1.3   Capitation

With capitation, the doctor is paid according to the *number of patients that
register with him or her* regardless of how much treatment they actually require
during a year. Capitation payments are suitable where the aim is to pay
doctors for providing health cover for patients rather than specific treatment.
This makes it an appropriate payment for general doctors working in
polyclinics who are given an annual payment in return for providing (first-
level) health care during the year. It is not usually suitable for specialists,
although hospitals may be paid the equivalent of a capitation fee to provide
in-patient care as necessary via a block contract (see section 5.2.1). Capitation
payments may be supplemented with appropriate fees for certain key
interventions but it is important that such additional fees do not dominate
other sources of income, otherwise the danger is that doctors will attempt to
earn these fees to the detriment of the rest of their work. This appears to be a
real danger in countries such as Hungary where the fee schedule for extra
work is long and quite complex.

The basic capitation payment may be *weighted* according to the needs of the
patient registering. Typically age and sex is taken into consideration since it is
well known that the young, the elderly and women of reproductive age
require more medical care, on average, than people in other groups. A more
sophisticated formula might take into account other factors, such as social
deprivation, which lead to greater ill-health. In the UK special payments are
made to GPs working in deprived inner city areas, measured according to an
index of variables which include housing, lone parents and proportion of
unemployed. Such payments are designed to compensate doctors for taking
higher need patients or working in higher need areas.

In the UK payment of GPs is complex. Around 60% of income is obtained
from capitation payments. The rest comes from a basic practice allowance
(salary element); special payments for looking after very young children; and
some fee for service target payment for achieving, for example, high levels of
immunisation coverage. A target income is set each year and capitation and
other payments adjusted so that this target is achieved by the average GP.

The incentives present with a capitation system are complex. The system
encourages doctors to compete for patients registered but, once registered, to

deliver as little care as possible. This is countered by the competitive process itself, which should lead patients to choose a GP who provides a good quality service. If a doctor fails to provide good treatment, then the patient always has the option of registering with another doctor.

There are two factors that may hinder this competitive process from working effectively. The first is that patients may judge a doctor not on the quality of medical treatment, which can be hard to measure, but on *easier (more superficial) criteria*, such as the quality of waiting facilities or the friendliness of the receptionist. In former Soviet Union countries a parallel may be the desire for sick-notes by patients. A doctor's readiness to sign such letters could be an important basis for the decision to register, regardless of his or her medical competence. This relates to the agency role of the doctor, and the fact that patients find it difficult to judge what they need and how they should obtain it. It is, however, a problem that should not be overstated for GP care, which is one part of the medical system with which patients have substantial contact.

A second factor is the *degree of competition* that operates between doctors. Although competition may be plentiful in areas where population density is high, in sparsely populated rural areas there is likely to be a lot less. An alternative doctor may be many kilometres away, rendering genuine choice and competition impossible. This problem is heightened if doctors join together in group practices. Although this has advantages in pooling overhead costs and allowing a more comprehensive service to be offered, it also means that doctors working together in an effective cartel reduce choice. In these circumstances, it is important that other forms of monitoring are in place. These include *medical audit* of different physician practices and the requirement for *regular re-registration* with a proper accreditation procedure.

An ever-present problem with systems based on capitation is *cream skimming*. Although in theory GPs may be forced to accept all that wish to register, in practice they may find ways of preventing high-need patients from doing so (see Chapter 2). Weighting payments for the main need factors such as age reduces this problem, but there will still be patients that are in low risk population groups but are high risk individuals. Informal mechanisms for dealing with such patients have sometimes been observed. For example, doctors in a village may agree to each register a patient for a six-month period, after which the patient is passed on to the next doctor.

5.2   PAYING HOSPITALS AND POLYCLINICS

There are a variety of ways in which contracts can be developed between the purchaser—health authority or insurance fund—and provider units. The aim of all should be to encourage efficient provision of quality services and delivery of the basic insured package. Contracts should encourage a range of delivery methods that permits wide consumer choice and equitable access to the basic package by all those insured. The next sections deal primarily with the incentive effects of various payment and contracting components. Chapter 7 will discuss the practical implications of these contract types.

5.2.1 Block or capitation contract

With block or capitation payment, a provider is contracted to deliver one or more services to a given population for a fixed sum per capita (i.e. per person). This type of contract can be used at different levels of the system:

- *First-level providers* (polyclinics and feldsher stations) to cover all ambulatory or primary care for a population during the course of a year.
- *Second-level providers* to cover services such as emergency care for the inhabitants of a certain area.

Two things should be noted. First, this contract effectively *transfers financial risk* from the insurer to the provider. Providers have to treat as many patients as come to them for the same level of funding. Secondly, there is an incentive for the provider to *reduce the amount of care provided* since it still gets the same payment.

It should also be clear that payment under the traditional Soviet system is a type of block contract. Providers receive the same level of funding no matter how much care is provided. The difference is that the contract is monitored for quality of care and, since the purchaser (insurer) is institutionally separate from the provider, it may move the contract if the quality is not high enough. If patients complain, for example, that some have been turned away, refused treatment, forced to pay extra or been given sub-standard service, the contract may be terminated.

An additional incentive for providers and an important way of increasing consumer choice are *individually determined capitation contracts*. In this case the individuals choose which provider to register with for treatment in the event of illness, for which the provider receives a fixed payment. Patients who are not satisfied can move their registration and the payment moves with them. A problem with this system (as with capitation at the primary level) is that providers may discourage patients that are high risk (the elderly for example) from registering. Even if they are not officially permitted to do this, they may circumvent regulations by, for example, siting their consulting rooms upstairs to discourage the infirm from registering. To avoid this behaviour and reward providers for a heavier volume of work, capitation payments are often weighted by risk factors such as age and sex.

Capitation payments may also be modified for other factors. For example, providers may be paid more for working in certain areas or offering 24-hour cover.

The effectiveness of individual choice will depend, as ever, on the availability of information with which to evaluate the provider, and the reality of competition between provider units in the area in which a given individual lives. With hospitals, there is the additional problem that patients may need to go to different hospitals for different types of treatment, and that quality can vary between departments within one hospital: the ear, nose and throat (ENT) department in one hospital may be excellent while the general medical department may be terrible.

In the US, the search for methods of cost containment (resulting from a combination of fee for service and third-party payment) has led to a proliferation of *health maintenance organisations* (HMOs), which provide total health cover for an individual for a fixed budget per year. This is a good example of a capitation system which, since it covers both primary and secondary care, gives incentives to bias services towards primary care, which is cheaper. This issue of *incentives to refer is important*. If the package of care is not carefully defined, GPs and hospitals will refer complicated cases elsewhere, thus reducing the costs to themselves.

5.2.2   Volume contracts

It may be more appropriate to *regulate the volume of some services* and pay accordingly. This is particularly true of elective surgery where the purchaser may wish to decide in advance the number of procedures to pay for. These contracts also carry less risk for providers. Volume contracts take advantage of the economies of scale achieved by providers when a large volume of one service is delivered. In this case the fixed or overhead costs (hospital running costs, nursing time etc.) become insignificant for each patient treated and the main cost elements are the marginal costs—theatre time and consumables. The purchaser specifies in advance the number of procedures it wishes to buy—for example, numbers of hernia or varicose vein operations. The provider is paid a sum for achieving this target, which will be less per operation than if each operation were purchased individually. The contract may also specify what happens if the volume is under- or over-achieved. The amount paid would be increased or reduced (within limits) but only by the marginal costs of the procedure.

Providers will need to *cost services* on a hospital or departmental basis for their own purposes in order to increase efficiency and determine what price will be required to cover costs. This is not the basis for pricing, however, which is the subject of negotiation between fund and provider. Providers should not be given higher prices for their services simply because their costs are higher (which would be an example of *perverse incentives*—i.e. where poor performance is rewarded rather than penalised). An oblast hospital gets no more for performing a normal delivery or appendectomy, for example, than a rayon hospital.

5.2.3 Fee for service

Fee for service is where a provider is paid for each unit of care delivered. A unit of care may be defined in various ways such as procedures given or patients treated. Payment will usually be received after treatment has been given but according to some pre-determined tariff agreed with the insurance fund.

There are a number of fee for service methods of payment that may be used.

5.2.3.1 *Length of stay*

In this method hospitals are paid according to the number of days (per diem) that a patient spends in hospital, multiplied by the standard daily charge, averaged over all patients or for some speciality. Until the mid-1980s this was the dominant method of payment for hospitals in countries with social insurance health funding, and it is still common today under voluntary insurance schemes. There is an automatic perverse incentive to *keep patients in hospital too long* since later days in hospital are generally much cheaper than earlier ones (involving recovery, rather than tests and interventions). Some countries have tried to counter this by paying a declining amount for each extra day above a certain level. This has generally not succeeded in reducing length of stay.

The rate per day (*daily charge*) is negotiated in advance between the payer and the participating hospital. The latter submits a report on the current and expected budget and number of patient-days. The expected budget is divided by the expected number of patient-days. The indicators used for projecting the budget can be either the hospital's prediction or the last available data, trended according to changes in the population, morbidity or the hospital's mission.

The insurer or rate regulator examines the utilisation of resources in the hospital by comparing the workload, length of stay, number of operations etc. with other hospitals. Deviations from the average serve as a signal for examining more deeply the performance of the hospital, with a view to adjusting the expected budget, number of patient-days and eventually the rate of daily charges.

The rates can be calculated in different forms:

- all-inclusive rates;
- rates for general services, but excluding some which are reimbursed separately at specific rates (e.g. maternity cases, the most complex surgery, some paraclinic services); or
- excluding the remuneration of doctors (who may be reimbursed using a fee for service method.

Some patients are more expensive than the average, and some are less expensive, but they should average out for the hospital as a whole. They should also average for each payer. If one sickness fund argues that it should pay less because its members require less intensive care, the method becomes unworkable.

The advantage of the method is in its simplicity. The main disadvantage is that hospitals have an incentive to encourage long stays. Monitoring costs are therefore incurred to ensure that hospitals do not abuse the system. In France, for example, the hospitals require licences from the sickness funds to prolong hospitalisation after the 20th day of stay. This is a relatively blunt instrument though.

5.2.3.2   Average cost

In this method daily charges are usually worked out on the basis of average cost. Alternatively, providers may receive a payment for each patient treated on the basis of average cost. This *rewards high cost providers* by paying more to expensive facilities and to facilities used less intensively. It does not encourage the efficient provision of health care.

5.2.3.3   Procedure-based cost

Here providers are paid for each procedure. There is an incentive to give each patient *too many tests or treatments*. This may be controlled to some extent by medical standards. The system also requires a complex system of costing that breaks down costs by each procedure given for each patient. In the Czech Republic, which operates a point system combining per diem payments with points for specific services, direct charges for materials and supplies are paid before any professional fees are covered. This feature, together with a valuation system which relates points to the time taken for each procedure, provides a bias towards invasive interventions (Massaro, 1994).

5.2.3.4 Medical economic standards

In this system providers are paid according to *disease diagnosis*. In each group patients must receive a certain protocol of treatment such as medication and diagnostic tests. The system requires a large initial set-up cost and the treatment given to each individual must be monitored from treatment records. This requires substantial resources, but may not be effective if the records submitted are inaccurate. The standard also defines which level of facility is able and allowed to perform each procedure. Prices are incorporated for each disease category. These may be hospital-specific or established as a national or local tariff.

5.2.3.5 Diagnosis-based cost

Here providers are paid according to diagnosis, corrected for severity, age and some secondary diagnoses and complications (*diagnosis related group—DRG—in the US; healthcare related groups in the UK*). Medical Economic Standards are the first step to defining a DRG-based system. As the price for each diagnosis is fixed in advance, there is an incentive to minimise the inputs into treatment, and, accordingly, when DRGs were introduced in the US, a reduction in average length of stay and total input use per case resulted (even though input per day increased). However, 'DRG creep' was found in the US in earlier systems, meaning that patients were assigned to more expensive categories simply by discovering a secondary diagnosis or complication. This problem has been reduced in later versions. There is also a potential problem of more expensive patients within given categories being referred elsewhere. Where the DRGs only apply to a category of treatments, for example, in-patient stays, then there may also be a shift towards interventions whose prices are uncontrolled (e.g. out-patient visits).

The main constraint, however, is the amount of information required by the DRG system—first to allocate patients to the right category using 'Grouper' software, and later to monitor to ensure that patients have been correctly grouped. There is also a balance to be struck between the administrative complexity of a large number of categories, and the incentives to select certain types of patients if there are fewer categories. There are high transactions costs, too, in billing procedures and the periodic renegotiation of reimbursement rates. On the other hand, the information on case-mix and costs has other uses, in terms of evaluating cost effectiveness of treatments and monitoring internal performance by the provider agencies themselves.

The DRG system is *prospective* in that the price of cases is set prior to treatment being given. This avoids the problems of retrospective payment where providers receive a larger payment simply by increasing the volume of treatment given. Since the payment is set, providers do not compete on the basis of prices but on volume and quality of service. A DRG or procedure tariff may be used as the initial basis for negotiation, but purchasers may then be able to negotiate block or volume deals for those they represent.

5.2.3.6   Target payments

This is a special type of fee for service often used in the primary health care setting, where a large but controlled volume of treatment is required as an indicator of the success of the programme. For example, providers may be paid for achieving high vaccination coverage and the payment may rise with the proportion covered. Providers cannot vaccinate more than 100% of the target population, and vaccination itself, provided it is administered correctly and the vaccines are in-date, is a good indicator of outcome. This contrasts with operations, for example, where simply operating on as many people as possible is no indicator of improved health status. Target payments may also be used for screening people for certain diseases—cervical or breast cancer, for example. They can be paid to primary providers in addition to capitation or other payments.

Using an econometric model of OECD countries, Gerdtham et al. (1992) analysed health service expenditures, using fee for service (FFS) payments in the out-patient sector as a dummy variable. Their results suggested an 11% increase in expenditures in OECD countries where the FFS method is widely used. This supports the a priori suggestion that FFS methods will increase levels of cost (and if cost per unit is fixed, by some system as described above, doctors can always compensate by increasing activity levels). Other studies suggest that providing care on a FFS basis costs one-third more than using capitation, without yielding substantial differences in health outcomes (Barr & Field, 1996). This may be the reason why global budgeting has returned to vogue in a number of OECD countries in recent years (Wolfe & Moran, 1993). There is also a clear consensus that retrospective reimbursement, using FFS— i.e. with no pre-agreed tariff, but charged at full cost after treatment has been given—is very unwise. Countries like Romania, which adopted this approach in their first wave of reform, are now looking for alternatives which facilitate cost control.

5.2.4   Fixed budgets

This is where a provider is paid a fixed budget per year, based on historical precedent usually, or on the basis of infrastructure or the number and type of people on the payroll. This last approach (staff-related fixed budgeting) is largely the method that operates in the former Soviet Union, with no separation between purchaser and provider (hence it is sometimes known as the *integrated approach*). Extra payment is achieved by employing more people which in turn may be determined by the number of (occupied) beds. There is therefore an incentive to *acquire more beds and staff*. The cheapest way to achieve this is to keep patients in hospital for long periods since treating more patients incurs additional costs. There is no incentive to provide good quality service, and where budgets are specified for different types of expenditure (*line budgeting*), there is limited managerial flexibility to plan and manage resources well.

However, *global budgeting* can be effective where it is based on more rational criteria, such as expected case-mix and utilisation of a hospital, and where management has the flexibility and capacity to reallocate resources to their most effective use. Australia, Norway and Portugal currently use this type of global budgeting for their hospitals (Barnum, Kutzin & Saxenian, 1995). Tight budget controls and quality control are important for the success of this approach.

Where global budgets are administered by teams of clinicians within hospitals, this is known as *clinical budgeting*. It aims to involve clinicians more directly in management decisions, such as the setting of performance targets, taking responsibility for working within budgets, increasing efficiency and raising standards of care. Incentives can be provided, in the form of retained savings from increased efficiency, for example. However, restructuring is usually required within the hospital to move from traditional departments to semi-independent budget-holding groups.

5.3 NOTE ON DIRECT USER PAYMENTS

A user payment is where the patient pays directly for services received. This is clearly an example of fee for service, but with the full brunt of the cost borne by the patient. The main advantage is that the user is less likely to abuse the system by demanding *unnecessary consultations* and treatment. In addition in some countries a patient may only believe the service is of high quality if such a payment is made.

The main disadvantages are that patients may be deterred from receiving necessary as well as unnecessary care and that the *poor are affected* by the payment more than the rich. Evidence from Western countries suggests that if used widely, user payment can have a detrimental effect on the level of effective treatment obtained as patients may be deterred from seeking vital first-level care, where diagnosis and subsequent referral occur. In addition, if the method of collection is complex, the *administrative costs* can quickly out-weigh any revenue generated from the payment.

It is most important that the *basic package* offered by the insurance system be free of any direct user payments. Patients should have easy access into the system through a first-level provider and then referral as appropriate and as the conditions of the insurance policy allow. If a patient is charged in addition, all credibility for the insurance system will disappear and individuals and enterprises will become unwilling to contribute.

Direct user payments might however be used in the following ways:

- charges for *self-referral* to second- and third-level providers for insured and non-insured patients;
- charges for all but emergency care for all those *not able to produce evidence of insurance cover*;
- charges for care that is provided *outside the basic package*—patients should be warned if the care is outside the package and given a detailed invoice of the amount to be paid;
- charges for *additional hotel services*—private room, fridge, tea-making, improved menu, business facilities—provided by the hospital. The costs of these services should be covered wholly by the patient; and
- charges for *drugs*, or part of drugs cost (to discourage over-use), or for drugs outside the basic list of essential drugs (to encourage cost-effective prescribing).

The scope for further cost recovery and income generation from direct payments should be explored by providers. The incentive to obtain income in this way will be increased if providers are given autonomy to manage the facilities themselves.

5.4   EVALUATION OF PAYMENT METHODS FOR INSTITUTIONS

Table 5.1 provides an evaluation of the different payment methods on the basis of the criteria established at the beginning of the chapter.

Capitation and volume contracts score highly since they are cheap to establish and require relatively little information to monitor. Cost containment is easy to maintain since payment is not directly affected by the amount of work done. The danger of too little treatment, which may reduce quality, may be limited by a requirement for basic information to allow comparisons between providers and departments and monitoring of patient satisfaction. These methods can be implemented with relatively little information and can be developed as the information base grows. For example, a hospital block contract may, over time, be divided into speciality contracts with some volume constraints.

Table 5.1 Evaluation of main payment methods, each ranked on the basis of scale 3 = good to 1 = poor

	Management cost	Cost containment	Incentive to be technically efficient	Impact on quality
1. Capitation				
First level (primary)	3	3	2–3	3
Secondary level	3	3	2	2
2. Volume contracts	2	2–3	3	2–3
3. Fee for service				
3.1 Length of stay	2	1	1	1
3.2 Average cost	2	1	1	1
3.3 Procedure-based cost	1	2	2	1
3.4 Medical economic standards	1	2	2	2
3.5 Diagnosis-based cost	1	2	2–3	3
3.6 Target payments[a]	3	2	3	2
4. Fixed budgets	3	3	1	1
5. Direct user payment[b]	1–3	2	1–3	2–3

[a] Use limited mainly to immunisation and screening.
[b] Evaluation depends on the way user payments are used.

Most *fee for service systems* require a large amount of information to monitor effectively and there is always the danger of excessive treatment. Each case must be monitored and controlled on an individual basis. In all cases it does not matter how complex the system of payment is, it will not function correctly if the methods of monitoring are less sophisticated. Fee for service systems vary in the extent to which they encourage technical efficiency.

Fee for service systems that are based on *length of stay* encourage long periods in hospital. Those based on the *average cost* of hospitals reward facilities for being inefficient. Where based on *number of procedures* too much treatment may be encouraged. The least efficient payment system would combine length of stay with average hospital cost per day treated.

Systems based on *medical standards* still tend to encourage patients to be kept in hospital up to the norm. They are complex to monitor and develop and tend to be based on average standards, which may not reflect best practice. Each case must be examined and penalties are paid if treatment given does not comply with standards.

Diagnosis-related groups can work effectively where information is plentiful and monitoring is well developed. They are expensive to develop and monitor and require a sophisticated system of costing already to be in place. The undeveloped nature of the management information system in many countries of the former Soviet bloc makes them unsuited to present conditions.

Fixed budget systems are easy to establish and monitor. There is little incentive to over-provide ineffective care but neither is there an incentive to provide effective care. There are no financial incentives to give quality service and these standards may have to be enforced in other ways, such as through medical standards.

Direct user payments, where used to reduce self-referral, pay for services outside the package and offer extra hotel services, can be a useful way of deterring unnecessary treatment and generating income. It may sometimes be difficult to collect money from patients, once treatment has been completed.

5.5 CONCLUSION: SEEKING AN OPTIMUM PAYMENT SYSTEM

Each payment system has its own strengths and weaknesses which must be balanced against those of the old system. In a general chapter it is not possible to make specific recommendations for all circumstances, since the ideal system will vary from country to country. Instead this final section will offer some general principles for a successful payment system.

Institutions
1. Payment systems have intrinsic characteristics but are also dependent on the *context* in which they are implemented. So, for example, paying doctors by capitation in one country may encourage doctors to improve services and permit patients to exercise greater choice. In another country it may simply encourage doctors to offer quick popular services such as a drugs prescription for every patient or a sick note to any person that asks.
2. The success of a system depends largely on the ability to *monitor its operation*. There is little point in introducing a case-based payment system if hospital statistics are not considered accurate or if the method of monitoring does not allow reliable verification of sub-department-level statistics.
3. A complex system may be counter productive if it impedes data being used for other purposes. If hospital staff spend all their time collecting data for the purposes of payment then they may be unable to focus on the *management role of financial information*. In addition, focusing on the average costs of individual departments or cases may deflect attention away from the way in which marginal costs react to changes in activity in that department or in other departments.
4. Even if the payment system is relatively simple, monitoring can still be sophisticated. It may be more effective to pay providers using an easily understandable and easy to administer system, but make longer term contracts contingent on a range of other *quality standards*.

5. It is important that providers use similar information systems to ensure *consistency in data quality*. A condition for payment might be that suitable systems are put in place.
6. Monitoring of *aggregate indicators* may be a more effective tool than attempting to regulate the treatment of every patient. Knowing whether a hospital has changed its overall performance in terms of peri-operative deaths, mix of cases or average length of stay can be more useful than trying to enforce rigid average standards on non-average patients.

Individual practitioners
7. It is important to *separate the method of paying institutions from the payment of individual practitioners*. Problems have arisen when the wages of medical staff are linked directly to payments received from an insurance fund or health administration. For example, if a hospital agrees to pay staff for patients treated for the insurance fund but the fund delays payment or later manages to negotiate a block discount with the hospital, the provider can be left with a heavy salary debt. Such a system also removes some responsibility from providers to determine the method and level of wage payments.
8. A related concept is that, in most cases, *payment to staff should not be directly linked to the amount of service provided*. There are a number of reasons, including that it:
    *   can lead to excess number of patients treated;
    *   penalises staff in departments not providing direct patient care, e.g. X-ray;
    *   concentrates attention on throughput of patients possibly to the detriment of other components of care (e.g. effective treatment).
9. A *broad range of indicators* should be used to monitor the performance of staff over a longer period of time on the basis, for example, of limited period contracts.

Payment systems, whether simple or sophisticated, can never be an alternative to effective planning. Experience all over the world suggests that even the most complex system can be exploited by providers. If the insurance fund uses a new payment system without properly understanding the effects of the system and the types of service that are really required, it is likely that the new system will produce minimal benefits for health. Indeed it may even be worse than the past system, since resources are used on more expensive administration and monitoring.

What is required is a carefully thought out strategy for planning and purchasing services that includes a suitable payment system, along with methods for assessing need and monitoring the system's effects and long-term impact on health status. These functions that should be performed by the purchaser of care are covered in greater detail in Chapter 4 on purchasing and Chapter 7 on contracting.

REFERENCES AND FURTHER READING

Barnum, H., Kutzin, J. & Saxenian, H. (1995) Incentives and provider payment methods. *International Journal of Health Planning and Management*, vol. 10, pp. 23–45.
Barr, D. & Field, M. (1996) The current state of health care in the former Soviet Union. *American Journal of Public Health*, vol. 86, no. 3, pp. 307–312.
Braham, R., Ron, A., Ruchlin, H., Hollenberg, J., Pompei, P. & Charlson, M. (1990) Diagnostic test restraint and the specialty consultation. *Journal of General Internal Medicine*, vol. 5, no. 2, pp. 95–103.
Donaldson, C. & Gerald, K. (1993) *Economics of health care financing*. London: Macmillan.
Gerdtham, U., Sogaard, J., Andersson, F. & Jonsson, B. (1992) An econometric analysis of health care expenditure: a cross-section study of the OECD countries. *Journal of Health Economics*, vol. 11, pp. 63–84.
d'Intignano, B. (1992) Health systems in flux as East meets West. *World Health Forum*, vol. 13, pp. 38–42.
Massaro, T., Nemec, J. & Kalman, I. (1994) Health system reform in the Czech Republic. *Journal of the American Medical Association*, vol. 271, no. 23, pp. 1870–1874.
Wolfe, P. & Moran, D. (1993) Global budgeting in the OECD countries. *Health Care Financing Review*, vol. 14, pp. 55–75.

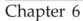

Chapter 6

PROVIDER PLANNING AND COSTING

James Piercy and Tim Ensor

6.1 WHY PLAN, WHY CHANGE?

The presumption behind most provider planning is that there is benefit in improving the quality and cost effectiveness of the services provided. In the Soviet-style system there were few general financial incentives to make changes although individual practitioners were fined for providing treatment that did not meet medical standards.

Even after a number of countries have implemented reform programmes it is often not clear why providers should wish to change. The pattern of services often reflects the one which existed prior to reform. Early financial incentives arising from new payment systems often appeared to encourage rather than diminish perverse behaviour (e.g. long lengths of stays encouraged by per diem payment). There are a number of reasons why a provider should change. These include:

1. *Ability to compete*: in the future health insurance funds will become more discriminating in what they want and do not want to purchase. A provider changing now will be in a better position to respond to these demands.
2. *Generate incentives for staff*: improving the cost effectiveness of services can release resources that enable providers to reward staff for implementing change.
3. *Improving the health of the population*: this should be the target for any public medical facility. Changing from normative funding towards patient-based systems enables providers to think in terms of patients treated rather than beds filled.

An Introduction to Health Economics for Eastern Europe and the Former Soviet Union.
Edited by Sophie Witter and Tim Ensor. © 1997 John Wiley & Sons, Ltd.

It is not possible in this short chapter to offer a complete description of the many ways in which the disciplines of health policy, management and economics might be used to engineer change within hospitals and polyclinics. For more detailed references the reader is referred to the further reading section. This chapter presents some basic techniques that might be used by a provider to assess current services and decide how these might be adapted in the future.

6.2 ASSESSING THE EXTERNAL AND INTERNAL ENVIRONMENT

The first part of a planning exercise is to assess the current level of services provided by the institution. To do this an inventory of current assets available in the hospital is required. This will include:

1. *Staffing*: numbers of staff; positions and vacancies; level of training; pay and incentives; current procedures for evaluating staff (if any).
2. *Physical facilities* (estate): age of buildings; state of repair; functional suitability and relationship of key departments to one another; maintenance inadequacies.
3. *Equipment*: quantity and description; age; state of repair and reliability.

Assembling these data often takes longer than initially anticipated. Ideally, to complete a thorough bed modelling or cost accounting exercise, data must be broken down by department. It is important to document data that are not available in order that procedures for collecting them in the future can be established.

Once an inventory has been completed the institution will need to review its own position as a provider of health care. To do this a technique often used is to document the *strengths* and *weaknesses* of the institution and also the *opportunities* that are likely to open up in the future and the *threats* from outside influences. This is known as *SWOT analysis*. An example of an opportunity could be the closure of another hospital that will bring more patients to the facility being assessed. An example of a threat might be where a polyclinic is considering offering a service on an out-patient basis that is offered by your hospital.

This review covers both the external and internal environment for the provider.

6.2.1 External environment

The provider might begin by focusing on the external demands for its services. These include demands made directly by patients for charged services

Table 6.1 Recognising potential opportunities and threats

Area	Aspects for examination: opportunities or threats
Strength of demand	Patterns of demand Changing demographic structure Changing needs of the population
Purchasers	Number and range of purchasers Purchaser funding and ability to buy services Changes in purchaser behaviour Potential dissatisfaction with current services
Competitors	Degree of competition Changes in services offered by neighbouring providers
Technological change	Ability to undertake new procedures
Political factors	Government directives Local and regional priorities Expectations of local population

and demands made by the public purchasers of medical care—the oblast health administration and/or the medical insurance fund. The assessment should look at likely changes in the patterns of services that will be required for patients in the future and examine the extent to which present facilities will be able to meet these demands. For example, if the population of the oblast is ageing then there will be greater demand in the future for treatments for diseases that increase with age such as chronic psychiatric conditions, strokes and cancers. Similarly there may be growing evidence that certain types of treatments do not work. In this case it is likely that purchasers will demand less of these services in the future. Other aspects related to this analysis are show in Table 6.1.

6.2.2 Internal environment

The second part of the analysis is to focus on internal strengths and weaknesses. Here the emphasis might be upon the way in which current services are provided. This might include areas such as human resources: is it becoming more difficult to retain skilled workers because of a developing private sector? Are the facilities arranged in a way that minimises distances that patients must be transported? Other aspects are shown in Table 6.2.

Once a general analysis of the facilities has been conducted then it will often be useful to conduct a more in-depth *review of individual departments*. This should involve both senior management—medical and economic—and senior

Table 6.2   Potential topics for internal analysis of areas of strength or weakness

Area	Aspects for examination: strengths or weaknesses
Human resources	Number of staff, retention, recruitment Training opportunities Working practices and internal communication Skill-mix
Facilities	Condition of the estate Functional suitability and appropriate space utilisation (using the estate wisely) Availability and condition of equipment Utilisation and appropriateness of equipment
Operations	Performance by specialty in terms of length of stay, outcomes, readmission rates etc. Range of services provided and clinical/specialty interdependence Patient satisfaction
Communications	Communication with purchasers and patients Internal communications between departments
Processes	Internal organisation/efficiency Clinical protocols Planning and administrative processes Ability to cost services accurately and methods of cost containment

members of staff from the department concerned. The aim will be to identify weaknesses in current provision and scope for future expansion. The departmental review might concentrate on the most common conditions (perhaps the top 10) and examine the way in which they are treated: most common method of treatment, overall length of stay in hospital, how long people wait for operations, how frequently patients have to be readmitted for the same condition etc.

6.3   PLANNING FUTURE SERVICES

The analysis of current service provision will begin to indicate those aspects of current services that require change. It is now necessary to explore the implications of these recommendations in a little more detail. To do this two interdependent modelling techniques can be used. The first is bed modelling which makes use of simple arithmetic relationships between occupancy, activity and length of time in hospital to model the effect of specific changes to patient workload. The second is a cost accounting system. Together they provide a powerful but adaptable way of measuring the impact of change.

6.3.1 Bed modelling

Bed modelling will usually be undertaken at a speciality or sub-specialty level. It requires information on *total activity* (numbers of admissions or deaths and discharges), *proportion of day cases* (if any), *average length of stay* and existing *number of beds*. All of these data should be readily available in hospital records.

From these data the total occupancy rate is given as:

$$\text{Occupancy rate} = \frac{\text{admissions} \times \text{length of stay}}{\text{beds} \times \text{available days per bed}}$$

Note that the number of days a bed is available each year varies considerably from country to country and often between rural and urban areas. It may be easier to assume all beds are available 365 days a year and then make some consistent and explicit allowance for cleaning and maintenance at a later stage.

Combining these data allows a manager to gauge the impact of a change in practice on the number of beds required. For example, perhaps it is found that the length of stay in a particular specialty is high (by national or international standards), perhaps because patients are kept in hospital unnecessarily or for simple changes in dressings that could be undertaken in an out-patient setting. Managers can use this formula to model the impact of reducing average length of stay on bed requirements in that ward.

More complex bed modelling will typically involve breaking down specialty activity into individual procedures or diagnoses. Individual lengths of stay can then be applied and the bed-days for each procedure calculated individually. The increased sensitivity allows the impact of technological change to be analysed on a procedure by procedure basis. For example, what is the impact on the bed and staff requirement (and total costs) of carrying out a surgical procedure such as gall-bladder removal using minimally invasive endoscopic techniques rather than a conventional open operation? Individual changes can then be taken into account by clinicians and managers when calculating the bed requirement.

As well as estimating the number of beds required, it is also important to estimate the number of *theatre sessions required*. Theatre modelling is based on future planned workload and should take into account demographic changes and any potential workload changes resulting from increasing or decreasing activity. It is important to consider the working arrangements of the provider, in particular the average number of cases per scheduled session.

Box 6.1   Example of specialty bed modelling

Assume that the average length of stay in a surgical department is 13 days, admissions are 1200 per year and there are initially 45 beds in a department. Bed occupancy (using 365 days per year) will be 95%.

Assume that a specialty review finds that people are being kept waiting in hospital for operations for an average of two days beyond what is necessary. If admissions could be managed so that this wait is cut the length of stay could be reduced. This would have some immediate effect on variable costs, for example, through a reduced requirement to feed patients. It would also lead to a decline in the bed occupancy to just 80% which could permit a reduction in the number of beds and staffing for the department. In our example, reducing the number of beds might lead to a new bed occupancy rate of 90%—still lower than it was before the changes occurred.

Box 6.2   Example: reducing length of stay in hospitals in Kazakstan

Increasing efficiency in hospitals implies reducing costs per patient treated to a minimum compatible with the desired standard of care. A recent study of hospital resource utilisation in Kazakstan (Ensor, Ryder & Thompson, 1996) focused on reducing the average length of stay (ALOS) for patients as a key strategy to permit a reduction in occupancy rates and then a reduction in bed numbers and restructuring of facilities, with the ultimate goal of making efficiency savings.

The first question was whether ALOS was in fact high. To answer this, ALOS in certain facilities was looked at, in terms of its trends over time, in comparison with other facilities with similar case-loads, and against the background of international trends.

The next issue was to find out why ALOS might be higher than necessary. A number of points emerged. First, payment systems are likely to influence ALOS. Paying per diem rates or rates based on actual costs is likely to increase ALOS. A possible solution would be to change to a case-based payment system or to pass on a proportion of efficiency savings to staff, although quality control would be needed if these were adopted.

Secondly, higher than average LOS might reflect the lack of resources, such as limited drugs supplies or anaesthesia to perform operations. Such bottlenecks could be alleviated by charging patients for specific inputs or by making efficiency savings in other areas and reinvesting them in such supplies.

Thirdly, medical technology might dictate longer LOS, where hospitals cannot afford to invest in equipment which permits swifter surgery and recovery times. However, it is equally possible that lack of familiarity with best international practice makes doctors unwilling to discharge patients, even where this is recognised as equally effective (and more cost effective). Managerial issues are also important, as there are many services which can be organised on an out-patient basis as long as adequate support facilities are available.

After considering the causes of high ALOS and possible solutions to these causes, providers should consider the likely impact on costs of reducing ALOS. Reducing ALOS alone will have only a small effect on costs, unless accompanied by more radical changes to the way in which hospital care is provided. For example, staff numbers could be reduced, which would have a significant impact on costs, and beds could be cut and facilities restructured to reduce fixed costs. In Kazakstan, it was estimated that up to 17% of the budget could be saved through ALOS and bed reductions. These savings could then either be passed on to purchasers or reinvested in identified priority areas, such as getting rid of shortages of key supplies, increasing salaries, or other investments in quality of services.

Table 6.3 Examples of hospital cost centres and types of costs

Services	Example	Fixed	Semi-variable	Variable
Direct	Cardiology	Heating	Nursing staff	Food and medicines
Paraclinic	X-ray	X-ray machines	Operators	Films
Support	Kitchen	Cooking equipment	Kitchen staff	Food
Overhead[a]	Administration	Computers	Secretaries	Paper

[a] Assumption is that variable costs relate to the total number of patients or patient days. Most activity in overhead departments will not be related in this way.

6.3.2   Costing systems

Costing systems have two principal uses. They can be used as a basis for pricing treatments to be used in contracts with purchasers. As important, although often neglected, they can be used in management decision-making. For example, costing systems might be used to work out the resource implications of the reduction in length of stay and number of beds suggested in the above bed modelling example.

The aim of a costing system is to allocate expenditure on the entire hospital to each patient department. There are several stages to this procedure.

First, *costs have to be allocated to each department or specialty.* Costs can be divided up in a number of ways. In addition to the distinction between fixed, semi-variable and variable costs, discussed in Chapter 3, costs must also be allocated according to whether they are directly attributable to a patient department, such as neurology or surgery, to a paraclinic department such as X-ray, to a support department such as laundry, or to an overhead department such as administration. These distinctions are illustrated in Table 6.3.

Items such as heating, lighting and maintenance will need to be allocated in an appropriate way as discussed in Chapter 3. For example, heating costs might be allocated according to the size of the building.

Once costs have been allocated to each department, the next stage is to *reallocate overhead, support and paraclinic expenditure to direct patient departments.* In doing this a step-down procedure is often adopted whereby overhead costs are first allocated to support, paraclinic and direct patient departments according to some common allocation factor. Support and paraclinic expenditure is then allocated to direct patient departments. Allocation often follows relative use made of each support/paraclinic department by patients. For example, X-ray expenditure can usually be allocated according to the number of X-rays performed for each department during a year. For more details on this step-down approach, see Drummond, Stoddart & Torrance (1987) and Dawson (1994).

Box 6.3 How to make a DRG

The following gives a summary of the main stages involved in dividing up clinical activity according to a case-mix-related workload (examples are based on 1985 groupings).

1. Divide all activity according to Main Diagnostic Categories (MDCs) derived from the International Classification of Diseases (ICD). For example, appendicitis and peptic ulcer would be classified into diseases and disorders of the digestive system.

2. Divide activity in each category into those requiring surgical and non-surgical intervention, e.g. appendicitis is surgical, peptic ulcer is non-surgical.

3. Divide surgical cases according to procedures; divide non-surgical cases according to main diagnosis.

4. Identify the main determinants of resource use within each of these categories using statistical techniques. Many systems have used the average length of stay as a proxy for resource use and then used cluster analysis (multivariate regression) to measure determinants such as age of patient and number and extent of complications. More sophisticated systems measure resource use in greater detail including, for example, amount of theatre time and nursing and doctor inputs.

Computer software (grouper software) is available to group cases automatically. A central part of this process is to exclude factors that make no difference to resource use. For example, age makes no difference to the average cost of treating a complicated peptic ulcer and so all cases are grouped regardless of age.

The final DRGs list the disease/procedure groups according to their relative resource use. In early versions of DRGs there were about 400 such groups, but later versions have increased the number. This compares with more than 5000 groups developed from medical standards reported in some Russian oblasts without the use of grouper procedures.

In the UK a system of healthcare resource groups (HRGs) has been developed along similar lines. The latest version was based on more than nine million hospital records and produced 528 HRGs. A considerable amount of effort and expense went in to developing the groups which must be updated regularly to reflect changing medical practice.

For more information see Bardsley, Coles & Jenkins (1989) and Sanderson, Anthony & Mountney (1995).

This procedure will give total expenditure by department and, by dividing by the number of patients treated annually or number of bed-days, a *cost per patient treated* and *cost per bed-day*. Two other refinements may be useful for planning and, later, pricing purposes. First, it may be useful to allow for *case-mix variation* since some patients in a department will be much more expensive to treat than others. Case-mix variation is the basis of various attempts at forming diagnostic-related groups (DRGs in the US; healthcare resource groups—HRGs—in the UK). The objective is to divide patients up according to main determinants of resource use, using the minimum number of categories possible. A general discussion of their advantages and disadvantages was given in Chapter 5. A summary of how they are created is given in Box 6.3.

A second refinement is to consider the *cost of a patient during the entire illness episode* rather than just while in hospital. This will usually be of more interest to a purchaser than a provider, but may be relevant if, for example, a hospital also provides some community services. For example, maternity care takes place in three stages: antenatal, intrapartum and postnatal. The total cost of an episode would include the time in hospital and also the cost of care provided in the community by midwives or doctors.

The resulting cost accounting model provides a description of current costs of services and will be useful for pricing purposes and comparisons between departments and hospitals. However, it can also be used dynamically to examine the impact of changing key parameters. The results of the initial situation analysis, bed modelling exercise and the cost accounting system can be integrated as a management tool for making decisions about future developments in the hospital. The costing model might be used to compute the implications of reducing the surgical length of stay suggested by the example in Box 6.1.

Another possibility is that the SWOT analysis might indicate that patients have to be moved a long distance when being transferred from the operating theatres to reanimation (intensive care) and then into the surgical departments. A reorganisation could make use of bed and costing models to work out the effect of alternative scenarios. Such exercises will also be useful as inputs into other management decision-making exercises such as option appraisals for new capital developments (see Chapter 8).

6.4   INFORMATION REQUIREMENTS

A major benefit of the planning exercise can be to realise what data might be useful for the on-going management of the institution. A by-product of many centrally planned systems (not just Soviet) was a proliferation of data collection forms and inventories that had to be filled in, often with little regard for their final use. As a result much information is collected and carefully stored but never used. This chapter has attempted to highlight how some of these data might be used in planning and management. It might be seen as a first stage in the development of a complete management information system (MIS) that links disparate data sets for management purposes. An important lesson is that, in order to collect data accurately and efficiently, staff must recognise that their collection serves an important function. Another lesson is that a complete system will require the co-operation and collaboration of a number of departments within the institution—accounting, economics, planning and medical statistics as well as individual departments—for it to function effectively. For more information on this important area, see Sheaff & Peel (1995).

6.5 MANPOWER PLANNING

As with facilities, the most important determinant of manpower requirement is the level and nature of activity. Once the projected activity is known, three crucial questions should be addressed:

- How many staff are needed?
- What type of staff are needed?
- When should they be recruited?

6.5.1 Number of staff

This is by far and away the most important issue for providers: the assessment of the number of hands required to undertake the necessary tasks. The key for the provider is to identify the *relationship between the volume of service and the capacity of staff to deliver it*—for example, how many nurses are required to provide care on a 24-bed ward?

This is not a simple relationship, since the standard or quality of service must be taken into account. There is a clear relationship (certainly in nursing) between the number of staff and the quality of service available. A ward, for example, could be staffed with a bare minimum of nurses, sufficient to ensure that only the most essential clinical tasks can be undertaken. On the other hand, if additional staff were made available, then a higher quality service would be provided. It is up to individual providers to decide what standard of care is to be offered, and thus determine the staffing requirement.

6.5.2 Type and grade of staff

Providers also face issues concerning the type and grade of staff to employ, and frequently they will have choices—for example, between nurses and support staff such as care assistants. Issues of skill-mix and potential substitution of staff may therefore be important.

However, *skill-mix* is perhaps not as important as commonly perceived, unless the relative differential in cost of staff in relation to the type of duties they are expected to perform is very substantial. It is far more important to get the numbers of staff correct, since substituting lower-grade staff typically does not make much difference to cost per case and is therefore simply playing at the margin. Relative differences in costs of salaries, in many parts of the former Soviet bloc, are likely to be small, and providers should not invest large amounts of time in fine-tuning the skill-mix.

6.5.3   Recruitment plan

The starting point for answering this question lies in the analysis of the current workforce. Providers should break down their staff into specific cohorts, defined by type (and possibly grade). They will then need to look at historic transition rates, that is:

- number of people leaving per year;
- number of people taking career breaks and returning to the workforce (e.g. pregnant women);
- rates of internal staff promotion;
- drop-out rates from training; and
- historical ability to recruit new staff.

It is then possible to project these factors into the future to estimate any particular recruitment and training requirements to balance any losses/gains with future changes in activity.

6.6   CONCLUSION

It sounds almost a tautology to suggest that managers of health facilities should look critically at their current activities, at the changes which may occur in future, and at the implications which these changes have for their future operations. Nevertheless, day-to-day survival is more often their focus than longer term planning. This is true not only in the former Soviet bloc, but elsewhere too.

Focusing on the gap between current and best practice, this chapter has outlined some simple ways in which managers can think about possible changes which might improve their activities and hence ultimately their survival as an institution. Although the examples have been taken from hospital situations, the techniques apply equally to the primary care sector. Situation analysis informs the modelling of staff, equipment and facilities needs. These in turn feed through into changing information requirements and human manpower planning and resulting cost implications. Information gained in these planning processes will also be useful when contracts are drawn up with purchasers. This is the theme of the next chapter.

REFERENCES AND FURTHER READING

Bardsley, M., Coles, J. & Jenkins, L. (1989) *DRGs and health care.* King Edward's Hospital Fund for London. 2nd edition.
Culyer, A. & Posnett, J. (1990) Hospital behaviour and competition, in Culyer, A.,

Maynard A. & Posnett, J. eds. *Competition in health care: reforming the NHS.* Basingstoke: Macmillan.

Dawson, D. (1994) *Costs and prices in the internal market.* York: Centre for Health Economics, Discussion Paper 115.

Dowie, R. (1991) *Patterns of hospital medical staffing: overview.* For the British Postgraduate Federation. London: HMSO.

Drummond, M., Stoddart, G. & Torrance, G. (1987) Methods for the economic evaluation of health care programmes. Oxford: Oxford University Press (see especially chapter 4: cost analysis).

Ensor, T., Ryder, S. & Thompson, R. (1996) *Hospital resource utilisation in Kazakstan.* Report for ODA Know How Fund, UK.

Green, A. (1992) *An introduction to health planning in developing countries.* Oxford: Oxford University Press.

Hutton, J. (1993) How providers should respond to purchasers' needs, in Drummond, M. and Maynard, A., eds. *Purchasing and providing cost-effective health care.* London: Churchill Livingstone.

Sanderson, H.F., Anthony, P. & Mountney, L.M. (1995) Healthcare resource groups— version 2. *Journal of Public Health Medicine,* vol. 17, no. 3, pp. 349–354.

Sheaff, R. & Peel, V. (1995) *Managing health information systems: an introduction.* Buckingham: Open University Press.

Sonenson, J. (1996) Multi-phased bed modelling. *Health Services Management Research,* vol. 9, pp. 61–67.

York Health Economics Consortium (1993) *Business planning for providers of health care services.* Harlow, Essex: Longman Group.

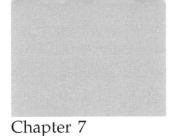

Chapter 7

CONTRACTING

James Piercy

7.1 INTRODUCTION

In any situation in which health facilities are not directly managed by health authorities, agreements must be reached by purchasers and providers as to what type, volume, quality and cost of health care is to be provided. This usually takes the form of some type of contract. This chapter sets out the basic principles of contracting, looking in particular at:

- the different types of contract available;
- the layout and structure of contracts;
- pricing and quality issues;
- content of contracts; and
- information requirements, monitoring and regulation.

The final section deals with the issue of contracting in situations where prices are fixed.

7.2 BASIC PRINCIPLES

7.2.1 What are contracts?

A contract is defined as a written (or spoken) agreement between two parties intended to be enforceable by law. Essentially, a contract is a statement of the rights and obligations of each party to a transaction. In the health care context, a basic example of a contract could be an agreement by a hospital to undertake 20 specified operations, for which it will receive (say) £20 000. Whether the money is paid in advance, after the work has been carried out, or in stages, is a matter for negotiation.

An Introduction to Health Economics for Eastern Europe and the Former Soviet Union.
Edited by Sophie Witter and Tim Ensor. © 1997 John Wiley & Sons, Ltd.

7.2.2   Basic elements of a contract in health care

Contracts in health care are largely between purchasers and providers, athough different providers may contract services from each other, notably in times of high demand or shortage of capacity. Purchasers include insurance companies, individuals, firms/businesses and the state. Providers include hospitals, polyclinics and individual physicians. However, all contracts would be expected to contain the same basic ingredients. These are:

- the nature of the work to be undertaken;
- the volume of the work to be undertaken;
- the price of the work;
- some specification of process (where relevant);
- information and contract monitoring; and
- legal issues relating to breach of contract etc.

Each of these will be discussed in more detail in later sections, apart from legal issues, which are very context-specific.

7.3   TYPES OF CONTRACT

In the health sector, there are three main types of contract available to purchasers and providers. These are block, cost–volume and cost per case. Each of these three types has advantages and disadvantages to purchasers and providers, and each can be appropriate in the right context.

7.3.1   Block contracts

A block contract exists where the purchaser pays an agreed fee in return for the opportunity to send any patients requiring treatment who fall within the scope of the contract. Hence, in theory, there is no restriction on activity. This type of contract is easy to arrange, and is often based on historical referral patterns. However, there is an implicit assumption made that referral rates and patterns are unlikely to change. To protect themselves against changes, providers may seek to impose a maximum limit on activity, and possibly some constraints on the type of activity.

For purchasers, block contracts are easy to operate, and guarantee a certain level of activity at a fixed price. However, a potential disadvantage is that they are inflexible where activity is lower than expected—for example, in maternity services, there might be fewer than anticipated deliveries or pregnancies. If this is the case, purchasers will spend more than strictly necessary.

Some form of under- and over-trading rules will need to be devised to ensure value for money is obtained (see Section 7.4).

For providers, block contracts have many advantages, not the least of which is guaranteed income to cover some or all of its specialty costs, regardless of actual workload. Such contracts allow providers to plan ahead how to meet the demand—for example, it can decide on an appropriate level of nurse staffing or an appropriate number of beds. The primary disadvantage is that providers do not receive any extra funding to cover extra workload. Equally, providers could be disadvantaged if case-mix is more complex than expected.

Block contracts are frequently used for emergency admissions, where demand is predictable and patients require immediate access to facilities. They are also useful for services such as maternity, again where demand can be estimated accurately, but less useful for elective activity, unless limits are imposed on overall volume.

7.3.2   Cost and volume contracts

In a cost and volume contract, the purchaser pays an agreed fee for a certain level of activity. Above that level, a cost-per-case deal is likely to be agreed. The activity level will be specified closely, e.g. £500 000 is paid for 500 pregnant women referred to the hospital. Occasionally, a 'tolerance' level will be built in, whereby purchasers will tolerate plus or minus a proportion (e.g. 5%) of the agreed activity without either penalising the provider or incurring extra costs. If the contract underperforms (i.e. there is insufficient activity), then purchasers will not necessarily be liable for the full value of the contract.

The primary advantage over a block contract for the purchaser is that they only pay for the workload they receive. However, a maximum activity level will need to be specified, or the purchaser could be faced with cost over-runs. This is particularly important if activity levels are rising. Given that providers are likely to cover their costs in a cost–volume contract (assuming all the anticipated workload materialises), purchasers may be able to negotiate for additional activity at a discounted rate, maybe even at marginal cost. This ability will depend on the relative importance of a purchaser to the provider. Health authorities and large insurance companies will be in a far better position to achieve this kind of deal than will individuals or small insurers/ practitioners.

Providers also see important advantages in cost–volume contracts if the volume is set high enough. Such contracts also usually guarantee minimum levels of activity, while avoiding problems if workload exceeds contract levels. It is also possible (if purchasers do not notice) to put low cost cases in the volume element and high cost cases in the cost-per-case element. The reason for this is that, in practice, only three-quarters of expected activity will be covered by the volume aspect, with the remainder being on a full cost-per-case basis up to the total activity agreement. Purchasers may wish to fix the cost element in advance (regardless of case-mix) in order to counteract this practice.

Cost–volume contracts are suitable for most health care contracts where demand can be estimated reasonably accurately. While they are not as straightforward as block contracts, they offer both purchasers and providers some flexibility around the margins, though it is important that the 'cost' element is negotiated carefully.

7.3.3   Cost-per-case contracts

The third key type of contract is cost per case. In this situation, the purchaser pays an agreed fee for each and every episode of activity. Each admission or contact is therefore covered by an individual contract. Such contracts are of most value when activity levels are small, uncertain or falling, since this contract type offers both purchaser and provider maximum flexibility.

Other than the inevitable higher level of transaction costs (these are the costs associated with negotiating the contract), cost per case allows purchasers maximum flexibility, particularly if they may wish to change referral patterns or are unsure about the quality of the provider. However, it will be difficult to negotiate discount deals linked to marginal costs; in a cost-per-case environment, purchasers are usually price-takers. The only exception to this may be for unusually complex referrals, where some negotiation may be possible.

In the UK, perhaps the most common use of the cost-per-case contract is in extra-contractual referrals. These typically occur in the following situations:

- complex referrals and tertiary referrals;
- where current providers reach capacity;
- emergency cases where the patient is away from home and referral to another (distant) hospital is necessary; and
- where small contract volumes are anticipated.

There are a number of advantages and disadvantages to providers. The biggest advantage is when providers have covered the bulk of their costs through routine contracts, and have a little spare capacity to undertake additional workload. Under such conditions, cost-per-case activity could be lucrative, particularly if there are no restrictions on prices. Given that purchasers are essentially price-takers in a cost-per-case scenario, negotiation costs to the provider may be lower than anticipated, as it may be possible to devise a 'standard' contract; inserting only the procedure to be carried out and the price as appropriate. The main disadvantage to the provider, other than the paperwork, is that there are no guarantees about volume and therefore about likely income. This can make planning more difficult and will generate considerable uncertainty, since costs tend largely to be fixed, at least in the short run. This is exacerbated if the main purchaser(s) operate on a cost-per-case basis.

7.3.4 Summary

As has been discussed, each of the three main contract types have advantages and disadvantages to both purchasers and providers. The choice of contract type will in practice be determined by:

- size of purchaser/provider;
- contract volume;
- ability to accurately predict volume; and
- nature of the referral.

Finally, it is worth noting that all contract types are available to all purchasers (except individuals who would naturally pay on a cost-per-case basis), in both the public and the private sectors, and to all providers of services. For further discussion of the incentives provided by different forms of contract and payment systems, see Chapter 5.

7.4 STRUCTURE OF A CONTRACT

All contracts except cost per case will have the same basic elements, regardless of the provider, the specialty concerned or the setting of the care. These elements include:

- period or duration of contract;
- services covered;
- volumes;
- quality of service;
- cost and payment schedules;
- information requirements; and
- renegotiation clauses.

In this section, each of the above will be discussed, with examples being drawn from both primary and hospital sectors as appropriate.

7.4.1   Duration of a contract

Typically, contracts will be set for the period of one year, though this can be extended or shortened if required. If contracts are for a longer time period, it may be necessary to include a renegotiation clause to cover unforeseen changes in activity, costs or the external environment.

It is also usual at this stage to identify what type of contract is being used, i.e. block, cost–volume or other, and whether this is likely to change over time. The type of contract is crucial as it influences the service specification, volumes, costs and payment schedules.

It is possible to set contracts without time limits, but simply for a given volume of activity. These are more awkward, and their practicality will be determined by factors such as provider capacity and payment method. If, for example, payment is up-front, or even as work is done, then providers may have incentives to delay provision of the service, especially if more lucrative opportunities arise. Contracts without time limits are not generally recommended.

Note that even though activity and cost will need to be negotiated annually, it is not unreasonable to devise a service specification in terms of quality, information requirements and monitoring arrangements to last for a number of contracts—possibly up to three or five years hence. Since detailed specifications are time-consuming to draw up, setting an on-going specification may be a way of reducing transaction costs. This only works, of course, if there is a stable relationship between purchaser and provider.

7.4.2   Services to be covered

The next task is to state what services will be covered by the contract. Depending on the nature of the service and the type of contract, this can be undertaken in differing amounts of detail. In maternity, for example, defining the service is straightforward, as episodes last from first antenatal visit through to last postnatal visit. Furthermore, the likely number of hospital admissions can be predicted with a fair degree of accuracy if contracts are on a sufficiently large scale (e.g. a couple of hundred episodes). It is equally possible to split contracts into hospital and community care without much difficulty, since maternity episodes would continue to be well-defined and self-contained.

In other specialties, specifying services is not so straightforward. In surgery, for example, the range of procedures is vast. If there is a lack of detail in service specifications, purchasers are vulnerable to providers undertaking primarily low-cost procedures (making excess profits in the process), while providers may have difficulties if purchasers refer large numbers of complex and expensive cases. In medicine, the majority of admissions are emergencies, so neither provider nor purchaser have much control over admission patterns. In this case, contracts need to be sufficiently flexible to ensure the purchaser only pays for activity undertaken, while providers are covered in case of excess workload or adverse case-mix.

One method is to contract by procedure (appropriate for surgery) and by diagnosis (for medicine). Previous experience and analysis of historical activity and treatment patterns will inform the provider and hopefully the purchaser about the relative cost of different cases, which can be reflected in the price of the treatment. Classification of cases can be a potential pitfall, though with the introduction of DRGs or HRGs (see Chapters 5 and 6), this should be less of a problem.

It is equally important to specify the nature of services in a primary care environment. In particular, issues such as diagnostic testing and responsibility for payment for pharmaceuticals need to be covered. If, for example, diagnostic testing is charged on a fee for service basis, purchasers have little control over costs while providers have clear incentives to provide additional (perhaps unnecessary) tests. In this case, contracts will need to contain agreed protocols about the level of service to be provided (see also section 7.4.4 on quality and section 7.4.6 on information requirements).

7.4.3   Contract volumes

The volume of service to be provided will vary according to the type of contract, but will always relate to the level of anticipated activity. In block contracts, the volume will relate to all expected activity, whereas in cost–volume some three-quarters of expected activity is likely to fall in the 'volume' element with the remainder covered by the 'cost' element.

A key decision that will have to be taken relates to the units by which the activity will be measured. The units of measurement are often referred to as the contract 'currency'. There are a number of ways of measuring activity, as outlined in Table 7.1.

Measuring activity in the health sector is notoriously difficult. Since it is largely impossible to measure outcomes, most activity monitoring focuses on process indicators, i.e. counting what has been done to (for) the patient, rather than what is the effectiveness of the care. In the UK, acute services are generally measured in terms of *finished consultant episodes* (FCEs). These represent the total time spent under the care of a particular senior specialist. This does not necessarily equate to time spent in hospital. For example, a maternity FCE would last from the first antenatal appointment, through delivery and up to

Table 7.1 Different possible currencies for contracts

Activity	Currency
Hospital in-patient	FCE Procedure Code
Hospital out-patient	Complete episode[a] Attendance Clinic session
Community nursing	Face-to-face contacts Caseload size Whole time equivalent
Community physician	Episode of care[a] Face-to-face contact Clinic session
Pathology	Request

[a] An 'episode' is defined as the initial attendance plus appropriate follow-up attendances.

the last postnatal visit. By contrast, if a patient changes specialist during a single admission, two FCEs will be recorded.

However, FCEs are not appropriate for all services—for example, for community services. Here, other forms of activity measurement (or currency) are more relevant. These include:

• face-to-face contacts;
• out-patient episodes or attendance;
• clinic sessions (e.g. for outreach clinics); and
• procedure codes (e.g. for day-case surgery).

Once a currency has been established, and a volume of activity agreed, contracts will need to take account of situations where the contract tolerance levels are exceeded. The tolerance reflects the variance of activity from an agreed amount that the purchaser is prepared to accept. This is important, since, due to the nature of the demand for health care and particularly when emergency situations are taken into consideration, activity cannot be predicted with absolute certainty. *Tolerance levels* of between 2% and 5% from intended activity are common in the British NHS, with the exact amount dependent on the service under consideration.

Where activity levels at the end of the contract period fall outside the specified tolerance levels, the situation of *under- or over-trading* occurs. If the contract underperforms (i.e. too few patients are treated), purchasers may be entitled to a refund or reduction in monies paid. For overperformance, the provider may be able to obtain additional payments, though probably at marginal cost. In all cases, rules need to be laid down in advance to cover these eventualities, particularly if block contracts are used.

7.4.4 Quality

Quality has a number of dimensions, and is difficult to define. Broadly, however, it relates to the style of services offered, ensuring that health care is delivered in a timely fashion and to an appropriate standard. There are two types of 'quality' that will be discussed here:

- outcomes; and
- patient experience.

7.4.4.1 Outcomes

Two types of outcomes are important: process outcomes and patient outcomes. The former relates to the method by which the treatment is carried out, the latter to the result of the treatment.

Process outcomes relate to the method of treatment. A key process outcome therefore is concerned with the establishment of *good clinical practice and treatment protocols*. These should be based on evidence of effectiveness wherever possible, though it is recognised that clinical judgements will also be important. The value of protocols is that they help to define pathways through the health care system, perhaps identifying appropriate diagnostic tests and investigations, hospital lengths of stay, criteria for invasive or medical treatment and appropriate use of day-case surgery. This should remove some uncertainty about potential increases in fee for service costs for the purchaser, while ensuring that the provider is able to meet appropriate (quality) standards. Wherever possible, protocols should be written or appended into contracts.

Patient outcomes relate to the success (or otherwise) of the treatment. Given that long-term outcomes such as success of surgical procedures are not usually going to be possible to monitor from year to year, other outcome measures are needed. Examples of possible outcome measures include:

- operative mortality (surgical cases);
- death before discharge (medical cases); and
- readmission rates.

7.4.4.2 Patient experience

A second measure of quality relates to the patient's experiences of care. Both hard and soft data could be valuable for quality monitoring. Hard data might include:

- waiting lists;
- waiting times in out-patients or in a surgery;
- ability of the provider to make and meet patient schedules (i.e. keeping to time);
- prompt arrival of discharge letter to the patient's own physician (important in a hospital context); and
- cancellation of appointments/non-attendance rates.

Soft data relates to issues such as:

- patient satisfaction with the care received;
- quality of the environment; and
- approachability/friendliness of provider staff.

7.4.5   Cost and payment schedules

A critical aspect of contracting relates to the payment of providers, in terms of both the level and the timing of payments. Regardless of contract type, it is essential to make the cost sections very explicit. Both parties need to know what amounts will be paid and when payment is due.

7.4.5.1   *What price is paid?*

There are two main issues: whether prices should be fixed for all providers or negotiated, and at what level—hospital, department, case—contract pricing should take place.

Simple pricing strategies often base prices paid to providers on the average costs of operating of each medical provider. Many newly developing insurance systems in the former Soviet bloc, for example, require hospitals to cost their services and then pay the average cost of providing one patient-day or treating one patient. As argued in Chapter 5, this rewards inefficiency by paying high cost providers more than low cost ones.

Two alternative options are available. The first is to fix prices across a number of providers. This may still allow scope for negotiation over volume but simplifies the overall process of setting prices. A possible strategy is outlined in Box 7.1. In this case non-price competition may assume a dominant role (see section 7.6).

A points-related system might be used in conjunction with a fixed overall budget to ensure that overall budgets are not exceeded (see section 5.1.2). In this case hospitals would receive relative payment according to the number and complexity of patients treated but the final payment would not be known until the end of the accounting period, when all treatment points are aggregated and divided into the total resources available. Cash advances provided

---

Box 7.1   Approach to fixed-price contracting in the former Soviet Union

1. Calculate the average cost per hospital admission for all hospitals in an oblast. For city and rayon hospitals use the average cost as the price. So, for example, if the unit costs for four rayon hospitals are 3000, 5000, 7500 and 10 000 tenge, the average would be 6375, which is the amount the fund would pay for each patient treated in the oblast.

2. If the unit cost is a long way above the average, the purchaser could begin paying more than the average but agree a plan with the hospital to gradually reduce the unit cost over a period of time.

3. Differences in case-mix may be reduced through a simple system of banding. Higher level hospitals might be placed in a higher band for payment purposes. So, for example, band one might include all rayon hospitals, band two oblast general hospitals and band three tertiary-level hospitals or national institutes.

4. These tariffs negotiated with hospitals should not prevent purchasers negotiating special rates with individual hospitals. An example of this is where a fund negotiates a lower rate per patient on condition that it sends a larger number of patients to this hospital. This type of contracting is likely to become more sophisticated over time.

5. The rates established in each oblast should apply to a volume of activity similar to previous years. If the number of patients exceeds a certain level the contract would specify that the hospital must agree a new level of payment. So, for example, the number of patients in a rayon hospital might be 10 000. Payment is made at 6375 tenge per patient, provided that last year's volume is not exceeded by 5% i.e. 10 500.

---

to hospitals would be adjusted once these values were known. The advantage is that good cost control over the entire budget is maintained. The disadvantage is that it involves substantial financial risk for providers. If the value of the point turns out to be much less than anticipated because all providers work particularly hard, then it may lead to financial difficulties. This suggests that even if such a system is effective in controlling costs on the purchaser side, some volume limits may still be required to reduce the financial risk to providers.

A second approach is to allow each hospital to negotiate contract prices with the purchaser. This has the advantage that hospitals are encouraged to reduce prices in order to compete but the contracting process is more complex and if there are few providers then the competitive process may fail to operate.

A compromise position is to use tariffs as a guide for contracting and as the maximum level of payment where negotiation proves impractical, but in addition to allow purchasers and providers to negotiate below these prices. So, for example, a hospital might be offered a contract that expands activity but only if a lower price per case is offered. Block discounts of this kind have advantages for purchasers, by using scarce resources for more patients, and also for providers since an expansion in activity can often be achieved at marginal costs that are well below average costs.

The second issue is the level of pricing. Initially an average cost per patient might be used as a basis for encouraging competition and giving purchasers a rough idea of relative efficiencies between institutions. Later, as information systems develop, costing and then pricing becomes feasible at a much lower level of aggregation. This may lead to specialty or department pricing and, eventually, diagnosis- or procedure-based systems (using, for example, DRGs). Although there are advantages in more detailed contracting systems, it is important that these do not exhaust the capability to monitor effectively or introduce an unacceptably high administrative cost (see Chapter 5).

7.4.5.2   When payment is due

The timing of payments will be crucial. There are three main options: payment in advance; payment after the activity has been completed; or payment in instalments. Providers would prefer payment in advance, whereas purchasers would prefer payment in arrears. However, in practice, neither may prove practical. Purchasers would be unlikely (unwise even) to pay the whole of the sum in advance, as providers may have reduced incentives to undertake the work to an appropriate quality or at the right time. On the other hand, payment in arrears could leave providers with cash-flow difficulties as salaries and other expenses have to be paid on an on-going basis. It is unlikely that providers would have sufficient working capital to allow this system to operate.

Payments are therefore likely to be staggered, and triggers for payment agreed in advance. Possible alternatives could be payment on a regular basis, maybe at the end of each month, or upon completion of certain levels of activity. That notwithstanding, it is likely that at least a portion of the payment would need to be in advance to avert cash-flow problems.

7.4.6   Information

Without monitoring, purchasers would have no idea whether they receive the activity they are paying for or when staggered payments might be due. Purchasers must ensure that information requirements are included in the contract, with penalties for non-provision of or late information.

Important information for contract monitoring purposes might include the following:

1.   In-patient hospital information
     • date of admission
     • department

- length of stay
- procedures undertaken
- diagnosis
- co-morbidities
- outcome
- admitting doctor
- residence of the patient
- age/sex information (of the patient)
2. Out-patient information
   - reason for consultation
   - tests or investigations performed
   - diagnosis
   - age/sex information
   - residence of the patient
   - first or follow-up attendance
3. Community/primary care
   - details of contact, e.g. who, where
   - tests or investigations performed
   - diagnosis, if appropriate
   - outcome of consultation
   - drugs prescribed
   - age/sex information
   - residence of the patient

Analysis by the purchaser might have a number of objectives such as:

- to examine the admission patterns of hospitals to see whether the case-mixes of patients change in response to changes in the payment methods;
- to audit outcomes of different hospitals and departments; and
- to provide essential information on changes in the pattern of disease within the region.

7.4.7 Renegotiation

There are a number of reasons that may lead to the requirement for contracts to be renegotiated. Many of these have been touched on already in this chapter, including:

- variations in activity levels, i.e. under- or over-trading;
- variations in costs of care;
- quality issues;
- lack of information;
- case-mix differences from the predicted activity mix; and
- changing demographic trends.

Contracts, particularly those lasting for a year or more, involving large sums of money or for a few (but complex) patients, will need to have renegotiation clauses, and triggers for the activation of such clauses.

7.5   DEVELOPMENT OF CONTRACTING

It is unreasonable to expect purchasers and providers to move from a system of direct management and state control of health care to a system with split purchasing and providing and expect elaborate contracts with detailed specifications to be drawn up instantaneously. In the first instance, assuming purchasers do not change referral practice, it is often sufficient to set a block contract based on historical activity for each specialty with prices to ensure that expected total hospital expenditure will be covered. The crucial point to note is that activity levels will need to be written into the contract to protect both sides from the problems of under- and over-trading and from case-mix difficulties.

Over time, as providers and purchasers become more familiar with the contracting process, higher levels of sophistication can be incorporated. These could include contracting by case-mix (DRGs or HRGs); cost–volume contracts with deals around marginal cost for additional activity; detailed quality specifications; agreements on waiting lists and waiting times for appointments; and maybe even including outcomes in the specification.

7.6   FIXED-PRICE CONTRACTING AND COMPETITION

In a free- or managed-market situation, provider units, be they hospitals or primary care physicians, will have to compete for business. In Western countries, the primary indicator is the price of the service offered, though other variables will also be taken into consideration by purchasers.

In competitive conditions where *prices are fixed*, purchasers are forced to rely on non-price indicators when choosing providers. Contracts will also have to be strengthened with regard to quality of service.

Factors which might influence purchaser decisions include:

- access to the hospital for patients (its geographical location and transport links);
- quality of care and reputation of lead clinicians;
- waiting lists;
- waiting time once at the unit;

- availability of diagnostic and treatment facilities including pharmaceuticals;
- quality of the environment;
- observed clinical outcome; and
- hospital efficiency and process indicators of performance (e.g. length of stay).

Under fixed-price competition and without subsidy, the only means providers have of ensuring financial viability is to attract sufficient workload to cover costs. The main means of attracting new business is for providers to offer a service at a higher level of quality than their competitors, offer more immediate access to care and be more efficient without compromising quality. The only alternative is to offer additional services to those set out in the minimum standard relating to the payment.

In a monopoly situation with fixed-price contracting, there will be little incentive for the provider either to cut costs or increase quality and acceptability of services. In this situation, the purchaser would be advised to encourage the development of alternative providers.

7.7 CONCLUSION

Contracting is a newly evolving art in health services which have moved away from an integrated system. It has to be sufficiently specific on important aspects such as quantity, quality and cost to allow clear understanding on both sides of the service to be delivered, while at the same time minimising the costs which are involved for both parties in establishing and monitoring the agreement. Similarly, a balance has to be struck between the interests of the purchaser in establishing a desirable pattern of care and incentives for efficiency and, on the other hand, the need for long-term planning by the provider and a stable market for their product. These skills are only just being established in many Western countries, and in the former Soviet bloc are at an even more elementary stage.

FURTHER READING

Atun, R. (1996) Why changing the contract currency can cut your bills. *Fundholding*, vol. 5, no. 1, pp. 24–25.
Atun, R. (1996) How to make sure you get what you pay for. *Fundholding*, vol. 5, no. 2, pp. 32–33.
Herd, A. (1995) How to get the best from your contracts. *Fundholding*, vol. 4, no. 20, pp. 28–31.

NHS Executive (1993) *National Steering Group on Costing for Contracting*. London: HMSO.

NHS Executive (1994) *Managing contracts: examples of further good practice and innovation in contracting*. Leeds: NHS Executive.

NHS Executive (1994) *Quality and contracting: taking the agenda forward*. Leeds: NHS Executive.

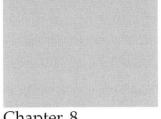

Chapter 8

OPTION APPRAISAL IN HEALTH CARE

Diana Sanderson

8.1 WHAT IS OPTION APPRAISAL?

Option appraisal has been defined (Mooney & Henderson, 1986) as:

> *a systematic examination of all the advantages and disadvantages of each practicable way of solving some problem or ameliorating some deficiency, with the purpose of promoting efficiency through informing rather than determining decisions.*

It is a logical and systematic approach which helps managers to make better decisions about changing the allocation and use of scarce resources. For example, investments in new facilities or new equipment often require considerable sums of capital, and thus have a high opportunity cost. The consequences of a poorly thought out decision will affect health care delivery for many years, so it is essential that these important decisions are reached only after well-informed local discussions. The option appraisal methodology ensures that decision-makers have relevant information arranged in an appropriate framework.

The ultimate aim of option appraisal is to *obtain better value for money* from limited resources, which is important irrespective of whether the capital for the investment comes from the public sector or the private sector. The benefits of option appraisal are summarised below:

- Helps to improve the clarity of defining the problem and setting the objectives by being *explicit* in considering the need for action.
- Gives greater appreciation of the advantages and disadvantages of alternative potential developments by being *systematic*.
- Helps to ensure that all aspects of a problem are given due consideration before the best solution is selected by being *comprehensive*.

An Introduction to Health Economics for Eastern Europe and the Former Soviet Union.
Edited by Sophie Witter and Tim Ensor. © 1997 John Wiley & Sons, Ltd.

Since the early 1980s, NHS hospitals in the United Kingdom have been required to carry out option appraisals before they bid for public money for capital developments. The NHS has issued guidance for this, which has been revised and refined several times. Since 1994 there has also been NHS guidance on assessing the use of private sector finance for capital developments. However, undertaking an option appraisal is an essential prerequisite to identify the most appropriate option to adopt. Much of the subsequent discussion of the methodology in this chapter is drawn from the most recently published NHS guidance (NHS Executive, 1994).

Although the discussion focuses on the steps that should be undertaken when considering a substantial capital investment, the methodology can be adapted for use in a variety of situations where smaller amounts of money are involved. The methodology can be used whenever decisions involving resources have to be made (e.g. acquiring a new piece of equipment such as a scanner or employing additional staff). It provides a good framework for ensuring that decisions are only made after the possibilities have been considered thoroughly.

8.2   WHAT ARE THE STEPS IN AN OPTION APPRAISAL?

The basic elements are listed below and described in the subsequent sections.

- Set strategic context
    ↓
- Identify objectives, criteria and constraints
    ↓
- Formulate long list of options
    ↓
- Reduce to short list of options
    ↓
- Assess and systematically compare costs and benefits of options
    ↓
- Consider uncertainties
    ↓
- Select preferred option

Before starting an option appraisal it is essential to identify *who will be involved* in its preparation. A small team (of four to six people) should be formed to manage and carry out the actual work, although its members should report regularly to more senior people within the hospital. The team should generally include people with clinical, managerial and financial skills, although this will depend upon the nature of the project. For example, building expertise will be needed to identify the relevant costs and timescales if the project requires comparing renovating an existing building with building a new one.

8.3   SETTING THE STRATEGIC CONTEXT

Before an option appraisal can be carried out, it is essential to examine the strategic context within which change is being considered. The seven steps recommended by the NHS (NHS Executive, 1994) are shown (with some modifications) below. They relate to the development of a new building, but can be adapted to other situations, such as the purchase of new equipment.

1. Consider past and future (local/national) health care trends.
2. Describe the current health care facilities and the benefits provided for patients.
3. Identify the likely future demand for the type of health care that will be provided in the facilities.
4. Consider the competitive position of the hospital/organisation.
5. Undertake SWOT analysis of the strengths and weaknesses (i.e. the internal capabilities) and the opportunities and threats (i.e. external and other trends) facing the organisation.
6. Identify the case for change, based on the gap between existing assets and future needs.
7. Identify the capital assets needs to meet future demand.

This part of the work is crucial, because it will provide the foundations for the subsequent work. For example, if we were considering the future provision of maternity services in a city, we would want to identify the relevant national trends and to examine local data on the use of current facilities. These might include: national and local trends in the birth rate; local population projections for women of child-bearing age for the next 10–20 years; how long women stay in hospital to give birth, and whether this is likely to change; whether national and local trends differ, and if so, why. It will be essential to identify the projected numbers of hospital births and the average lengths of stay before the required bed numbers can be determined, plus all of the necessary supporting facilities (e.g. operating theatres for caesarian sections; neonatal intensive care cots). Without this information it will be impossible to identify the size of the facility that will be required to meet future needs.

It is also important to consider the market in which the hospital/organisation is working. Are there any local competitors (e.g. for standard surgical procedures)? Who will purchase the service that you are considering providing, and do they want to purchase it? For example, there might be a need for more dialysis machines in a city, but if health insurance companies and other purchasers are not willing to buy additional dialysis sessions (e.g. because they give a higher priority to other types of health care), then there is no market for this service at present.

Depending upon the size of the project, this part of the work may take up to six months. However, it is time well spent if it prevents poor, ill-informed decisions from being taken.

8.4   IDENTIFY OBJECTIVES, CRITERIA AND CONSTRAINTS

Two types of *objectives* need to be identified—the broad objectives of the organisation and the specific objectives of the investment. The organisation's broad objectives should flow from national strategy and policy aims. They may simply take the form of a broad *'mission statement'*, such as 'the hospital wishes to provide high quality, accessible care in appropriate facilities, using well-trained, motivated staff and modern equipment'.

The specific investment objectives should relate to the outcomes that are required from the project. Investment objectives should be SMART—*specific; measurable; achievable; relevant; and with a time element* (see the list below). Good objectives not only refer to 'improving', 'reducing' or 'maintaining' activity, but also specify quantifiable targets (e.g. to reduce energy usage by 15% within five years). It is important to remember that the investment objectives should focus on the 'ends', and not on the 'means' for achieving these. Therefore, for example, if the hospital laundry is unable to meet current demands due to using poor quality, old-fashioned equipment which keeps breaking down, the objective is not 'to replace the existing equipment with new machines', but rather 'to ensure that the hospital can launder x items per week with a turnaround of y days or less'. There are many ways that this can be achieved, which might include paying another hospital or private company to do the laundry.

It is essential to identify at the outset what is to be achieved, because the objectives form the benchmarks against which the options are assessed. If you do not know what it is that you wish to achieve, it is impossible to determine whether or not a particular option meets your requirements!

The *criteria* lay out in more detail the expectations of what will be achieved in meeting the objective. They form a link between the objectives and the options, in that they can be used to judge the suitability of the latter to meet the former. Criteria should meet the conditions shown below.

- Criteria must be clear, explicit and well-defined.
- Criteria must be independent.
- Criteria should be quantifiable if possible.
- 'Good' performance must be unambiguously agreed.

Criteria must be defined and agreed, and it is particularly important to identify the conditions under which a particular option will score well against each criterion. For example, ground-floor accommodation with access to an enclosed play area provides a better environment for the care of sick children than the 10th floor of a building. It is also important not to double count by having dependent, overlapping criteria. For example, does 'accessibility' only include accessibility for patients and their visitors, or does it include accessibility for staff? If it includes both of these, then accessibility for staff should not also be included under 'ease of attracting and retaining high quality staff'. Some possible criteria are presented below. It is important to use only criteria that are relevant to the particular project. Between five and ten should be selected—any less and a criterion will catch too many opposing influences, and any more tend to be too cumbersome.

- Quantity of service (e.g. numbers of beds; numbers of patients; numbers of episodes of care).
- Quality of service (very hard to quantify, so need to identify proxies such as range of support services available, or range of specialties/sub-specialties available).
- Quality of buildings (need to consider their physical condition, functional suitability, and their external environment).
- Accessibility (generally for patients and their visitors).
- Ease of recruiting and retaining high quality staff (it may be necessary to consider the different types of staff separately).
- Ease of management (it may be harder to manage a service on several sites rather than on a single site).
- Acceptability (there may be several strands here, such as acceptability to users and acceptability to local residents).
- Ease of achievement (this considers how long it will take to deliver the option, and how easy or difficult this is expected to be).
- Flexibility for futue use (health needs are likely to change over the life of a building—can it be adated for other uses?)

Finally, it will be necessary to identify any genuinely binding *constraints*, such as a site of insufficient size or a location where planning permission would not be granted for a building of more than a specified height. However, beware of people who favour a particular solution stating that other options are not possible for various reasons. These constraints may turn out after further consideration to be genuine, but they may not!

8.5   FORMULATE LONG LIST OF OPTIONS

There is an art to formulating the long list of options, for this requires taking ideas from as many people as possible and combining them into a coherent list of possibilities. Long lists should be imaginative and exhaustive. They avoid myths about constraints and ensure that all possible solutions are considered. Long lists should include a wide range of possibilities, as shown below:

- A baseline option for comparison (the 'do nothing' option).
- A 'do minimum' option (which may be the same as the baseline option).
- A 'Rolls-Royce' option (top quality, ignoring all financial 'constraints').
- 'Politically' important options.
- A full range of alternatives, which may include counter-intuitive options.

Experience suggests that the best way to generate a long list of options is to have a *'brainstorming' session*. This will need to be chaired by someone with authority, who must spell out the ground-rules at the start and ensure that they are kept. The aim of the brainstorming is to get everyone's ideas (however odd they may seem) on ways of meeting the investment objectives. It is vitally important to invite all key players to attend—do not be tempted to exclude a particular person who is known to be awkward and difficult. Indeed, it is especially important to invite such people along, not only because they often have good ideas, but also because if they are involved at this stage they cannot latter complain that they have been ignored. They are much more likely to co-operate throughout the option appraisal exercise if they have been encouraged to contribute their ideas. The two main ground rules are that everyone should be encouraged to give their suggestions, and that nobody is allowed to criticise anyone else's ideas. Often ideas that initially seem inappropriate turn out to be quite inspired. Timid or less senior staff may have some excellent ideas, but may be reluctant to voice these if they feel that they might be ridiculed by other colleagues. Therefore strong but sympathetic chairing is essential. In addition, someone needs to write down all of the ideas that are generated, so that none are forgotten.

Unfortunately, the brainstorming session will not provide the long list. Instead, it will simply provide a wide variety of ideas which will need to be drawn up into a coherent list. It may be possible to identify groups of similar ideas—such as suggestions for the location of a new facility, or ideas about the scope of care that can be provided in hospital or in the community (e.g. mental health care). In the case of relatively straightforward option appraisals, the long list may only include a few options (e.g. if considering options for providing hospital laundry services), but in more complex situations the long list may extend to over 100 options. It is important to group options into options and sub-options wherever possible, since this will make it easier to identify the short list.

8.6 REDUCE TO SHORT LIST OF OPTIONS

There are a number of ways to do this, but a relatively easy way is to compare each option with the current (i.e. baseline) situation using the agreed criteria, especially if the options can be sub-divided (e.g. by location and by scope). For example, if there are several possible locations, these can be compared with the current location with regard to criteria such as accessibility for patients and visitors and appropriateness of the environment. Options which are outperformed by the baseline option against several of the criteria should be rejected, as should options which are outperformed by other ones. The aim is to reduce the long list to a short list of about five options that cover the broad spectrum of possibilities.

The short list must include either the 'do nothing' option (i.e. continue exactly as at present) or the 'do minimum' option (e.g. undertake essential repairs) as the baseline for comparing the other possibilities. Costs should not be considered at this stage, for they are examined in detail for the short-listed options. Reasons for rejecting options should be recorded in case this information is needed in the future. In fact, it is important to record the reasons underlying decisions throughout the process, for it is often necessary to return to these to justify decisions that have been made.

8.7 ASSESS AND SYSTEMATICALLY COMPARE COSTS AND BENEFITS OF OPTIONS

Once the short list has been identified, it is necessary to identify and compare the benefits and costs associated with each option. Weighted benefit scores are calculated for each option. This involves two stages—*weighting the criteria* and *scoring the options*. The criteria are weighted to reflect their relative importance. This is inevitably a subjective exercise, and can most easily be achieved by giving key people a list of the criteria (plus their definitions) and asking them to allocate 100 points across the criteria. Individual allocations can then be averaged to give an overall weight for each criterion. Scoring the options should be a more objective exercise, and is best performed by a group of people. Each short-listed option is assessed against each criterion, and given a mark between 0 (could not be worse) and 10 (could not be better). The scores for each option are then multiplied by the criteria weights and added to give *weighted benefit scores* for each option. Table 8.1 provides an example.

In order to compare the costs it is necessary to calculate the *net present value* of each option, discounting the costs over an appropriate period (see Chapter 3 for details about discounting). For example, a new building may be expected to last for 60 years, and should therefore be discounted over this period, whereas a piece of equipment may only be expected to be used for, say, five

Table 8.1 Calculating the weighted benefit score

Criteria	Weights	Option 1		Option 2		Option 3		Option 4		Option 5	
		Score	WS	Score	WS	Score	WS	Score	WS	Score	WS
Accessibility (patients)	25	3	75	4	100	9	225	9	225	7	175
Appropriateness of location	20	4	80	6	120	8	160	9	180	8	160
Ease of staffing	15	4	60	5	75	7	105	9	135	5	75
Ease of management	5	2	10	7	35	4	20	6	30	9	45
Flexibility	10	4	40	6	60	9	90	7	70	8	80
Acceptability	20	2	40	8	160	6	120	9	180	6	120
Time to implement	5	8	40	6	30	5	25	5	25	8	40
Total	100		345		580		745		845		695

years. It is also important to identify the time profiles and phasing of developments (e.g. of buildings), since these will affect the net present values. Some options may initially involve considerable capital investment (e.g. a new heating system), but will deliver substantial revenue savings over their lifetime. Discounting over too short a period will not reflect these long-term cost savings to the hospital. If items (e.g. a computer system or a building) are discounted over shorter periods than their expected lifespan, their residual value at the end of the period under consideration must be included.

Costs for each option (as positive values) are generally broken down into capital, revenue and land costs, with any income (e.g. from land sales) being included as a negative value. All costs should be stated against an agreed base year (i.e. general inflation should not be taken into account, although costs should be adjusted if they are expected to rise/fall at a different rate from general inflation). If the development is to be funded from public money, the discount rate should reflect the rate of return that would be achieved if the money were invested in government stock. However, if it is to be funded from money raised by the private sector, then the commercial rate, which is usually higher, should be used.

Table 8.2 shows the calculation of the net present value for a piece of equipment discounted at 6% (the current rate used in the NHS in the UK) over a five-year period. The equipment is assumed to have depreciated by 75% of its initial value at the end of the period. The first option, Option A, is the baseline and shows the cost of repairing the current piece of equipment (which is assumed to be fully depreciated), plus the annual revenue costs associated with its operation. The second option, Option B, purchases a relatively cheap new piece of equipment, which costs less to run each year than

Table 8.2 Calculation of net present values for three options

(a) *Actual costs*

	Option A			Option B			Option C		
Year	Cap.	Rev.	Total	Cap.	Rev.	Total	Cap.	Rev.	Total
1	1250	600	1850	2500	350	2850	4000	200	4200
2		600	600		350	350		200	200
3		600	600		350	350		200	200
4		600	600		350	350		200	200
5		600	600		350	350		200	200
6					−625	−625	−1000		−1000
TUC	1250	3000	4250	1875	1750	3625	3000	1000	4000

TUC = total undiscounted costs.

(b) *Discounted costs*

		Option A			Option B			Option C		
Year	DR (6%)	Cap.	Rev.	Total	Cap.	Rev.	Total	Cap.	Rev.	Total
1	1.0	1250	600	1850	2500	350	2850	4000	200	4200
2	0.943	0	566	566	0	330	330	0	189	189
3	0.89	0	534	534	0	311	311	0	178	178
4	0.84	0	504	504	0	294	294	0	168	168
5	0.792	0	475	475	0	277	277	0	158	158
6	0.747	0	0	0	−467	0	−467	−747	0	−747
NPV		1250	2679	3929	2033	1563	3596	3253	893	4146

NPV = net present value.
Discount rate (DR) = $1/(1+r)^n$ where r = discount rate and n = number of years.

the current piece. The third option, Option C, uses a more expensive piece of equipment which reduces revenue costs considerably. With these capital and revenue costs, Option B has the lowest net present value and Option C has the highest.

8.8 CONSIDER UNCERTAINTIES

Before deciding which is the preferred option, it is essential to consider any uncertainties and risks associated with the options. For example, does an option depend upon something which is entirely outside the control of the organisation, such as a land sale? If so, what would the effect be if the sale did not proceed, or if the sale only raised half of the expected amount? What would happen if wage costs rose or fell? An option which relies heavily upon staff rather than buildings/equipment will look considerably less (more)

Table 8.3 Comparing the costs and benefits

	Option 1	Option 2	Option 3	Option 4	Option 5
Weighted benefit scores	345	580	745	845	695
Net present values of costs	791	995	1424	1100	1002

attractive if wages increase faster (slower) than the costs associated with the buildings and equipment. What happens if the criteria weights are changed—does this affect the weighted benefit scores enough to alter their ranking of the options?

8.9 SELECT PREFERRED OPTION

The preferred option is initially identified from a comparison of the costs and the benefits associated with the various options. These are best set out in the form of a table, such as Table 8.3.

When faced with such a table, a few decisions can be made easily. For example, Option 3 can be rejected because it offers fewer benefits than Option 4, but costs considerably more. Option 3 is the only one that can be rejected because it is outperformed by a cheaper one. However, comparison of Options 2 and 5 suggests that Option 2 should also be rejected, since it conveys considerably fewer benefits than Option 5, but is only marginally cheaper. This leaves three options for further consideration, and there is no 'right' or 'wrong' preferred option. For example, Option 4 may be associated with considerable risks or uncertainty, and these may be felt to be unacceptable. Furthermore, although Option 4 conveys the most benefits, it is the most expensive, and purchasers may not be willing to pay this amount.

If it is still not possible to identify the preferred option after such considera-tion, it is necessary to compare the additional benefits that will be gained for the additional expenditure, and to decide which is the most appropriate option to adopt. For example, if Option 4 has been rejected because it is felt to be too risky, do the extra benefits of Option 5 compared with Option 1 justify the extra expenditure? Option 5 delivers twice as many benefits for a 25% increase in costs. It can also be useful to return to the weighted benefit scores table at this stage, since this shows exactly where a particular option is superior or inferior to another.

Undertaking an option appraisal will not always unambiguously identify the most appropriate option, but it will help to inform the decision-making process.

8.10   CONCLUSION

The option appraisal process outlined above will not make decisions for you, but it will help you to identify and assess the various possible ways of achieving your objectives and of delivering more cost-effective health care from scarce resources. Initially it may seem a cumbersome and time-consuming process, but in reality it provides a rigorous and disciplined way of approaching problems and of finding appropriate solutions. It is crucial to keep detailed records of all decisions, and of the reasons underlying them, so that it is possible to explain, for example, why certain options were rejected and why costs were calculated in a particular way. A short report should also be written, outlining each stage. This will enable other people to see how and why the preferred option was selected, and will also provide a benchmark so that actual performance can be compared with expected outcomes. It may also encourage others to adopt the same approach to complex decision-making.

REFERENCES

Mooney, G. & Henderson, J. (1986) Option appraisal in the UK National Health Service. *Financial Accountability and Management*, vol. 2, no. 3, pp. 187–202.
NHS Executive (1994) *Capital investment manual: business case guide*. London: HMSO.

Chapter 9

THE PRIVATE SECTOR AND 'PRIVATISATION' IN HEALTH

Sophie Witter and Igor Sheiman

9.1 INTRODUCTION

The idea of privatisation of health facilities is fashionable in many countries. Advocates of privatisation argue that it can enable health systems to get better value for money as a result of more cost-effective, innovative and responsive performance. In Russia and Eastern Europe the impulse to develop the private sector is stronger than in the West, as a result of their recent history and the distrust of state control and regulation which this has bred. Privatisation, of funding as well as provision of health, is regarded by many as the cornerstone of any health reform.

Institutional support for such a development in the former Soviet bloc comes from medical staff and organisations in particular. The best hospitals and medical research centres whose services are in demand are eager to attain the legal status of enterprise, which would enable them to decrease their commitment to the public system, choose the range of services provided and set their own prices. Private funding is also seen as a vital source of additional revenue and thus of income for health professionals.

This chapter will look briefly at different possible combinations of public and private sector finance and provision, and will then go on to examine what it means to be a 'private' organisation. What does experience from the West and from the former Soviet bloc in recent years suggest about the relative strengths of public and private sectors? The chapter looks in some detail at recent developments in self-governing status in the UK and Russia. It goes on to conclude that the public/private distinction often obscures more than it reveals, and that it is the regulatory and managerial frameworks which are more important in affecting the behaviour of organisations

An Introduction to Health Economics for Eastern Europe and the Former Soviet Union.
Edited by Sophie Witter and Tim Ensor. © 1997 John Wiley & Sons, Ltd.

Table 9.1   Public/private finance and provision

	Public finance	Private finance
Public provision	NHS (UK)	Copayments User charges
Private provision	GP in NHS Contracted-out support services	Private insurance

9.2   PUBLIC/PRIVATE MATRIX

Both finance and provision of medical care can be public and private, or a mixture of both. The interaction between different modes of finance and provision are illustrated in a simplified form in Table 9.1.

In the UK, as in the former Soviet bloc, most medical care is provided by state-owned medical institutions, and financed from public sources— primarily from central and local budgets. The major distinction between them is that in the former Soviet bloc the bulk of primary care is provided by state-owned polyclinics, which employ both primary care providers (district physicians responsible for serving a specified area) and specialists, most of whom render specialist care on an ambulatory basis.

In the UK and most other Western countries, primary care is separated from secondary care (financially and operationally) and is provided by private free-standing general practitioners. They contract to health authorities (HAs) to supply a specified volume of care to a registered population. So this is an example of public finance and private provision.

Another example of public finance for private provision relates to hospital support services, for example laundering, cleaning and catering. By using competitive tendering and contracts for specific services, hospitals may be able to make cost savings and/or get a better quality of service than if they used their own staff.

Similarly, private finance can fund private providers, as in countries like the US with predominantly private insurance and privately owned facilities, or it can be used to increase income in the public sector through user charges or copayments for medical treatments.

Chapter 2 on funding health services listed some of the problems relating to access and hence effectiveness of health services if private finance is the main source of funding. Even user charges as a top-up source are controversial because of the blunt nature of demand management: as well as limiting demand for 'unnecessary' treatments they can discourage poorer families from seeking essential treatments. At the same time, they do not necessarily control costs, as they can encourage physicians to provide services which generate revenue, whether appropriate or not. In China, for example, investment in high-technology equipment is popular in (public) hospitals as a way of circumventing the government's price controls on more basic tests and treatments. The administrative costs of collecting user charges can also often be high in relation to the revenue generated.

This chapter will therefore focus more on the supply side, so powerful in the health field, and in particular on the status of provider facilities and how this may affect the pattern of services provided.

9.3   MEANING OF 'PRIVATE'

It would be easy if we could go on to list the characteristics of the private sector and compare them with the strengths and weaknesses of the public sector. However, on closer inspection the meaning of these labels becomes increasingly unclear. More than one dimension needs to be considered.

9.3.1   Management of provision

One dimension of privatisation is the move from centrally controlled management of facilities to a situation in which local managers have the ability to control factors of production and levels of production. Although this is often thought of as decentralisation rather than privatisation, it nevertheless can produce profit-maximising behaviour of the kind generally associated with private ownership. In China and Vietnam, for example, land reform centred around restoring control over production to the peasants, which resulted in a surge in production despite the fact that land continued to be owned by the state (Ensor, 1996).

The type of management freedoms which may be extended in a period of transition from central direction include:

- the ability to shift resources between budget lines;
- the ability to set overall budgets;
- raising and retaining revenue;
- setting or supplementing wages;
- hiring and firing staff;
- purchasing equipment;
- selling buildings and retaining part or all of the proceeds;

- freedom to go bankrupt, or, in the case of a management team, to be fired for failing to meet objectives or making a loss over a given period; and
- right to select mix of services provided.

Most former Soviet bloc countries have introduced some of these managerial reforms, but few have introduced all. In particular, allowing providers to go bankrupt is controversial, given their political profile and the need for market stability.

In Russia as in the UK, a class of providers is being developed, termed 'non-commercial organisations', which remain within public sector ownership and are subject to some government restrictions, but which are given wide managerial freedoms. This attempt to combine the advantages of private-sector-style management with the advantages of public control will be discussed further below.

9.3.2   Distribution of profits

Another dimension is the regulation of profits and their use. A hospital or polyclinic may be constituted in a number of ways. For example:

- no surplus may be earned;
- surplus to be used in the development of facilities;
- surplus to be used to supplement wages;
- surplus to be divided between staff; or
- surplus to be divided between shareholders (which could be private or could be the state and/or staff).

Thus, for example, many of the 'private' hospitals in the US are non-profit-making, while many public facilities in transitional economies, especially in more affluent areas, are starting to make and keep surpluses. These are often subject to government regulation, but these regulations may not be fully enforced.

9.3.3   Ownership of facilities

A third dimension is ownership, or the right to sell capital stock such as land and buildings and use the money for other purposes. This is what is usually considered to constitute privatisation. However, it should be clear by now that the public/private divide is by no means so clear cut. For example, in the United Kingdom, the self-governing hospital trusts, while still in the public sector, have been given some ability to dispose of assets, while maintaining essential services to the public.

9.4   PRIVATE FUNDING AND ITS INFLUENCE ON PROVIDER BEHAVIOUR

A significant trend in countries which have recently legitimised private payments to public facilities is what can be called *'privatisation from within'* or *'creeping privatisation'* (see Smithson, 1993, and Ensor, 1996). Although facilities remain in the public domain and funding continues to come from the public sector, the control which once was linked to that funding is weakened by the erosion of the value of public sector salaries relative to the incomes to be made in the private sector. This is true of countries like China and Vietnam, but also of a number of former Soviet bloc countries where a lively private sector economy has developed.

In this situation, provider institutions orient themselves to maximising income from private sources, either through drug sales, formal user charges or the less clear-cut expectation of 'presents' in return for a decent standard of service, or any service at all. This in turn affects the pattern of services—not only in terms of affordability, but also encouraging the more lucrative activities at the expense of possibly more effective ones (this is particularly true of preventive activities and family planning, which are often relatively unprofitable). It becomes more difficult for the government to control health policy in this case, despite management links with provider institutions. At the same time it is often more difficult for the institutions themselves to control staff, who may be engaged in a number of profit-making activities, such as running private clinics in the afternoons or out-of-hours.

Rather than allowing privatisation to occur *de facto* and without government involvement, it may be preferable for self-governing institutions to be developed within the public domain, operating within clear and enforced rules about charging, exemptions, priority for public health services and use of surpluses. To do so, however, will require re-gaining control over funding sources, for example through the establishment of social insurance.

9.5   RELATIVE PERFORMANCE OF PUBLIC AND PRIVATE PROVIDERS

Theory would lead us to expect that providers at the 'private' end of the spectrum are profit-maximisers. This in turn suggests various characteristics, such as innovation, efficiency in use of inputs, and responsiveness to consumer demands. At the same time, we would expect them to concentrate on the most profitable services, to avoid socially disadvantaged groups with greatest health needs, and, when a third party is paying, to compete on quality rather than price.

So while the private provider offers *potential gains in technical efficiency*, it is by no means sure that allocative efficiency will be positively affected or that overall cost control will be facilitated. The extent to which gains in technical efficiency are made will also depend on the *market environment*—i.e. whether close competitors exist, how prices are regulated, and whether factor markets are liberalised so that input prices and volumes can be varied by management. Competition is usually limited to certain parts of the market, such as elective surgery in hospitals and diagnostic procedures, with little competition over emergency services, for example.

Empirical studies looking at the impact of ownership of hospitals have had to control for differences in case-mix size etc. and their results vary between studies (see Donaldson & Gerald, 1993, chapter 8). However, the general conclusion is that for-profit hospitals do not necessarily operate more efficiently than not-for-profit ones (i.e. their costs and prices are often higher) and their quality of service and outcomes are not consistently higher either. Moreover, there is some evidence that cream skimming does occur—i.e. that private hospitals (both in the USA and Australia) take less severe cases, leaving the more severe ones to be dealt with by public hospitals.

Evidence from the growing private sector in Eastern Europe tends to support these conclusions. In the Czech Republic, for example, where the ranks of private doctors are growing rapidly, charges to insurance companies are on average 10% higher for private care than state polyclinic services (Massaro, Nemec & Kalman, 1994). Initial data suggest that private doctors both perform more procedures and charge a relatively higher cost per case. Patients are more likely to visit more often—10 times per year, rather than an average of six for state employees. Earnings in the private sector are therefore much higher—usually at least twice that of the public sector. It is not yet clear what the effect on quality of care has been though.

In summary, private ownership is likely to lead to increased competition and efficiency only if the market is structured and regulated appropriately (and in those conditions better performance could also have been expected from public facilities). The impact of private ownership on equity would, other things being equal, be expected to be negative, although again this will depend on how health care is being financed and how prices are set for services.

9.6   SELF-GOVERNING STATUS

The concept of self-governing status for providers has gained popularity in countries which used to depend heavily on the integrated model of health care. Its underlying aims are:

- To grant providers *new freedoms in managing* the production of health care services, but not to the degree of complete commercialisation of their performance. They are to remain in the public system and be controlled in terms of the services they provide, quality requirements, and sometimes the prices charged for their services;
- To create *competitive pressures* and increase technical efficiency in a regulated market of medical care by granting purchasers the power to purchase services from a number of providers, using a contracting system based on agreed volume, cost and quality.

To achieve this, assets are handed over to the provider to dispose of subject to certain limitations, such as:

- maintaining a specified range of services;
- using income from these and any supplementary activities for costs and reinvestment rather than dividends to stockholders;
- establishing a board of directors which includes both non-executive directors, who represent the wider community, and executive directors, who carry out day-to-day managerial work;
- in return for accepting these limitations, they may enjoy some privileges such as tax exemptions or credits; and
- if for some reason the entity ceased to exist, the assets would return to public control.

9.6.1   Experience in the United Kingdom

By 1996 almost all NHS providers of non-primary health care (hospitals, community services and ambulances) had become self-governing trusts, selling services to health authorities, GP fundholders, private patients, insurance companies or other trust hospitals.

Hospitals are responsible for 'core' services in their area: emergency care; immediate admissions to hospital from emergency departments including emergency surgery; other acute cases which require immediate admission; out-patient and other services which are needed in support of the first three categories; and also public health activities, including services for the elderly and mentally ill, district nursing and health visiting. Other services (such as elective surgery, which patients can wait and travel for) can be sold under competitive bidding to other purchasers.

NHS Trusts are constituted as public corporations. They are given an interest-bearing debt equal to the value of initial assets and are free to dispose of their assets subject to exceptional intervention of the Secretary of State (Minister of Health) if a disposal does not comply with the mission of the hospital. The main condition for achieving self-governing status is that the management of the hospital has to demonstrate the skills and capacity to run the hospital, including sufficient information systems.

What has been the effect of these new trusts? It is hard to make definite conclusions after such a short period of implementation, which also coincides with a number of other changes which can serve as explanatory factors. Initial impressions are that *activity rates have increased*, although whether this is linked to a positive trend in outcomes is another matter. The power relationship with GPs has also changed, largely as a result of the creation of GP fundholders whose money hospitals now have to seek to attract. On the negative side, there are concerns about *increases in the cost of management* under the new system (hence calls for 'more white coats and fewer grey suits') as well as instability in the market and the difficulty of planning services under this more fragmented system.

9.6.2 Russian experience

In Russia the first steps towards self-governing status were made in the process of implementing the 'new economic mechanism in health care' (NEM) which was adopted by the government of the former USSR in 1989. Providers were given new powers in decision-making of which the most important were:

1. the right to establish the pay rates for the staff within the specified portion of provider's income devoted to payroll; and
2. the power to supply services to the private sector (industry and consumers) at negotiated prices.

In many regions of the Russian Federation, the integrated model of relationship with HAs has given way to a contractual one. In three regions (Leningrad, Kererovo and Kuibishev) polyclinics have become fundholders, receiving funding from HAs on a capitation basis and paying for each referral to hospitals for in-patient care, out-patient services, diagnostic tests and emergency calls.

They remain directly managed by HAs, though, with a lot of limitations on their performance. They have to comply with specifications relating to the area they serve, the volume and types of services provided, the percentage of income which can be used to pay staff and to reinvest etc. Cross-boundary flows of services are limited and subject to the authorisation of HAs.

Most regions still pay hospitals according to bed capacity and number of staff, while the majority of polyclinics are paid according to the number of patient visits and staff. This is a very distorting indicator, and some experiments with DRGs and capitation are now under way. However, the notion of direct management will be further challenged by reforms in the way in which health care is funded, especially if health insurance becomes dominant.

An option which is being discussed now is to introduce three types of legal status of providers with different powers and degrees of separation from HAs:

1. *State-owned directly managed providers.* HAs keep control over their operational performance, specify the area served, the volume and structure of services, management structures, pay and other conditions of employment. Hospitals and polyclinics with this status are committed to serving the local community and providing emergency services, psychiatric services etc. They are budgeted by HAs from the central and local budget.
2. *Private for-profit medical enterprises.* These work according to the law on 'Enterprises and entrepreneurial activity' which regulates the private sector. Commercial firms are not obliged to have any commitments to the public health system. If they choose to have any under mandatory health insurance they have to join the General Tariff Agreement and sell services at regulated prices.
3. *State-owned and private non-commercial organisations (NCOs).* They remain in the public health system but become self-governing entities enjoying the right to sell their services to different purchasers within the limits imposed by the government. They will be responsible for their own affairs without intervention from health authorities.

All three types of providers will compete for public money, but it is possible that with their combination of entrepreneurial incentives but underlying public accountability, NCOs will eventually dominate the health market.

Note that in Russia the origin of NCO status lies not with providers previously owned by the state, but with the medical facilities which in the past used to belong to state industrial enterprises. Most state-owned enterprises used to have their own 'medsanchast' to serve employees and the local population, and these would automatically have become private under economic reforms. The creation of the NCO was therefore necessary to prevent them becoming fully commercialised in their aims and activities.

9.7   CONCLUSION

The public/private distinction in health is not so much the clear-cut matrix presented in Table 9.1 as a spectrum, and a spectrum which has more than one dimension. Starting with the issue of provision, we need to ask a number of questions:

- How much control do managers have over day-to-day managerial decisions?
- Who has the right to sell assets and re-deploy resources?
- Who controls the surplus, if a surplus is generated?

We also need to consider the sources of funding, as these affect the behaviour of providers.

- What is the balance between funds raised directly from private individuals (including private insurance) and funds raised from publicly controlled channels?

The further along the various axes an institution is, the more it is likely to exhibit profit-maximising tendencies, on the one hand, or to be subject to state control on the other. However, beyond that we have also to consider the regulatory and general social framework within which the provider exists. Providers at most points along the spectrum will respond to the incentives set by different payment systems, the way in which the market is structured, the number of competitors, the availability of information about performance, and quality and price controls. There is no inherent superiority of private over public—or indeed vice versa. We return then to the themes which have been running through this book as the key determinants of supplier behaviour.

One of the important features of the trend towards increasing autonomy for providers, be they nominally public or private in nature, is the *changing role for central government* which is implied. Instead of being a micro-manager of facilities, it becomes a market regulator, charged with accrediting facilities, licensing doctors, setting public goals in health and putting incentives in place to encourage both purchasers and providers to meet them. Whether the facilities are public or private, it requires new skills and investment to regulate them effectively, both of which are still lacking in the former Soviet bloc. This changing role will be discussed more in the final chapter of the book.

REFERENCES AND FURTHER READING

Donaldson, C. & Gerald, K. (1993) *Economics of health care financing*. London: Macmillan.

Ensor, T. (1996) *Health sector reform in Asian transition countries*. Draft report for Asian Development Bank, Manila.

Massaro, T., Nemec, J. & Kalman, M. (1994) Health system reform in the Czech Republic. *Journal of American Medical Association*, vol. 271, no. 23, pp. 1870–1874.

Smithson, P. (1993) *Health financing in Vietnam: sustainability case study*. London: Report for Save the Children Fund (UK).

Part V

CONCLUSION

Chapter 10

HEALTH REFORM IN EASTERN EUROPE AND THE FORMER SOVIET UNION

Tim Ensor and Sophie Witter

In this final chapter we look at some of the major trends in health reform in the former Soviet Union and Eastern Europe in order to focus on the main lessons for future health system development, followed by a brief overview of some of the points raised by this book.

10.1 HEALTH STATUS IN THE FORMER SOVIET BLOC: A CENTURY OF ACHIEVEMENT, A DECADE OF FAILURE?

Recent health trends in pre- and post-communist former Soviet bloc (FSB) countries show some deterioration. Most indicators of health status lag well behind those of established market economies (EMEs). Infant mortality in Russia is 2.5 times that in EMEs, while in the Central Asian republics the factor is more than four times. The current disease profile in the FSB is an uncomfortable mix of first and third world. Rates of cardiovascular disease and neoplasms are rising, yet at the same time a number of infectious diseases, such as diphtheria and tuberculosis, are beginning to re-establish themselves as major health problems. It is not surprising that most countries look, usually to the West, for radical solutions to these endemic problems.

When looking at recent history it is easy to forget the considerable improvements made in the health status of the population since the beginning of the century. Before the outbreak of the First World War the death rate in Russia was more than double that in England and Wales, while the infant mortality rate exceeded 270 compared to less than 150 in England (Hyde, 1974; Fraser, 1984). By 1930 infant mortality had been reduced to 140—a trend that continued into the 1960s when the figure was comparable to that in England and

An Introduction to Health Economics for Eastern Europe and the Former Soviet Union.
Edited by Sophie Witter and Tim Ensor. © 1997 John Wiley & Sons, Ltd.

Infant Mortality Rate

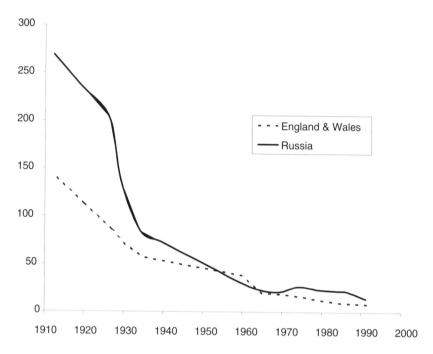

Figure 10.1 Twentieth-century trends in infant mortality in England/Wales and Russia

Wales (see Figure 10.1). It is only since the 1970s that this trend has shown some reversal.

The substantial reduction in mortality in Russia could largely be attributed to the virtual eradication of a number of infectious diseases such as malaria, rickets and polio (Hyde, 1974; Mezentseva & Rimachevskaya, 1990; Rowland & Telyukov, 1991). Also significant was the improvement in housing conditions. Similar gains were obtained in other FSB countries.

In recent years the most prominent feature of these countries then is not the absolute levels of mortality and morbidity, which compare quite favourably with other middle income countries (see Table 10.1) or the substantial ground made up since the First World War. Rather it is the trend in indicators that have remained stagnant or deteriorated while in most other middle income or EME countries statistics have improved.

The challenge for any reform process is to attempt to correct the imperfections of the past system while at the same time keeping the positive features. The

Table 10.1 Key indicators for Eastern Europe and the Former Soviet Union (data from *World Development Report*, 1996 and *Social Indicators of Development*, 1995)

	Income per capita ($US)	Infant mortality rate	Life expectancy[a] (years)	Doctors per 10 000	Beds per 10 000	Illiteracy (% of 15+)
Armenia	660	21	73/6	38.3	83	1
Georgia	580	19	73/8.2	54.9	105	1
Tajikistan	470	47	70/5.6	23.0	70	2
Albania	340	29	72/5.8	14.0	40	<1
Low income[b]	380	63	62/2.1	1.5	10	41
Azerbaijan	730	28	71/7.9	39.1	104	3
Kazakstan	1560	29	70/8.8	39.5	133	3
Kyrgyzstan	850	34	69/7.7	32.3	106	3
Latvia	2010	14	69/11.6	35.6	120	<1
Lithuania	1320	13	70/11.1	42.9	127	<1
Moldova	1060	25	67/8.1	39.5	123	4
Russian Federation	2340	21	67/11.9	45.5	137	2
Turkmenistan	1390	56	65/6.9	36.0	118	2
Ukraine	2210	16	69/9.9	44.6	132	2
Uzbekistan	970	40	69/6.1	35.6	95	3
Bulgaria	1140	14	71/7.1	31.4	96	<1
Czech Republic	2710	9	71/7.1	36.8	82	<1
Poland	2260	15	71/9	22.2	56	<1
Romania	1140	23	70/6.7	18.7	79	<1
Slovakia	1950	12	71/8.9	35.0	909	
Turkey	2970	62	67/4.1	10.2	25	12
Lower middle income[b]	1590	39	67/5.9	3.1	17	19
Belarus	2870	16	70/10.6	43.1	127	2
Estonia	3080	16	69/11	39.2	95	<1
Hungary	3350	15	69/9.3	30.3	103	<1
Slovenia	6490	8	73/9.8			<1
Upper middle income[b]	4350	36	69/5.9		25	14
High income[b]	23 680	7	77/6.4	22.1	69	<1

[a] Overall life expectancy followed by difference between male and female life expectancy.
[b] Italic rows are the world averages for countries in each income band.

reduction in mortality was a product of intensive attempts to provide basic health care to the population, particularly through mass vaccination campaigns. There is a danger that, in the scramble to introduce decentralised market structures, these very significant achievements of central planning are lost. A recent demographic and health survey in Kazakstan, for example, found that only 44% of children had received all three doses of the DPT (diphtheria, pertussis and tetanus) vaccine. This is a significant reduction on earlier years and in fact is much lower that many middle and low income countries.

Before reviewing some of the major reforms occurring in the FSB, it is useful to define some of the positive and negative features of the past system. This gives a better idea of what problems the current change process is attempting to address. Important features included the following:

1. Funding for the health sector was derived almost exclusively from state revenue sources. The overall cost of administration was probably quite low, total expenditure was easy to control and central planning ensured that a similar pattern of services was available throughout the Soviet Union.
2. All health facilities were owned and run by the state. Funding was provided to health facilities, based on fixed norms. Management in health facilities had little control over activities and inputs.
3. A network of rural facilities—feldsher stations, ambulatory clinics and rural hospitals, often supported by state farms—permitted access to the entire population. The high coverage and emphasis on prevention ensured that each person had contact with a medical practitioner on a regular basis.
4. The effect of Soviet-style central planning was to place great emphasis on input indicators such as numbers of doctors and hospital beds. Over time these became disassociated from indicators of need such as size of the population.
5. Consequently the level of medical infrastructure is high relative to established market/high income economies and very high compared to middle income countries. Much of the FSB had more than 40 doctors per 10 000 population.
6. Salaries of medical workers in FSB countries have been historically low and have got lower during the transition process. In Russia, for example, wages in 1980 were 75% of the average wage and by 1990 they had fallen to 68%.
7. A specialist culture made it unpopular to become a general physician dispensing first-level care. Those doctors working at this level often had inferior training and were less well equipped.
8. This culture meant that many major specialties had their own hospital at the oblast level of government. Hospitals received a high level of funding and rural and ambulatory treatment tended to lose out.

Together these features led to a health system that was considerably more sophisticated and integrated than is usual for an upper middle income country. It is notable that some middle income countries such as Turkey (see Table 10.1), a comparable country both in income and population diversity, are still struggling to develop a universal funding system. A central weakness of the system was that financial allocations were essentially passive, determined by the level of physical infrastructure. This meant that financial planning could not be used as a way to direct and improve the efficiency of systems through incentives. It also meant that as overall resources diminished the response of the system was to spread them more thinly rather than restructure capacity.

10.2   HEALTH SYSTEM CHANGE DURING TRANSITION

The process of economic reform has exacerbated some of the existing deficiencies of the system as well as introducing some new problems. It has led to a change process in the health sector that is in part driven by the type of reforms conducted in the economy, in part reacting to the effects of the economic changes and in part driven by ideas originating outside the FSB (e.g. driven by donors such as the World Bank). A number of common themes are apparent in this process.

10.2.1   Funding health care: mainly a question of more money?

Paramount among concerns is the desire to obtain more money for the health sector. State expenditure certainly fell in real terms and as a proportion of GDP in most countries just before and since transition started. This is largely the result of deep economic recession that has swept across Eastern Europe and on into Russia. Transfers from state enterprises, the traditional source of government income, declined, yet new sources such as profit and turnover taxes have not yet developed sufficiently to replace lost revenue. As a result state budgetary revenues have suffered disproportionately as a result of restructuring of the economy. Across the former Soviet Union government revenue fell from an average of 35% of GDP to 25% between 1991 and 1995.

A consequence of the reduction in state revenue was a general decline in the allocation for the health sector. Spending has never been high in any FSU country by OECD standards, although it has been comparable to most middle income countries. Extremely large health care infrastructure undoubtably means that resources are spread more thinly.

Medical insurance is seen as a way of obtaining an earmarked source of revenue that could significantly increase overall funding for the health sector. One view of this process is that if additional resources are forthcoming then many of the health system problems will be resolved. This analysis is flawed in at least three respects.

First, the discussion in Chapter 2 suggests that obtaining significant additional revenue will not be easy. An additional payroll tax is mainly aimed at formal industrial, frequently state, employment. It may not be easy to introduce in countries where the rate of urbanisation is low, as in many of the Central Asian countries, for example. In addition payroll contributions tax enterprises at a time when many are already overburdened with tax and are often unable to meet the costs of their operations. As the structure of employment continues to change this form of contribution may get harder to obtain. An illustration of these factors is Kazakstan, which began operating a compulsory scheme at the beginning of 1996. Two problems were apparent by the end of the year. First, many enterprises were unable or unwilling to make the payment and actual contributions were running at only about 25% of expected. Second, as many as 25% of the population outside the workforce or working in self-employment were not covered by insurance. In Russia, by the end of 1994, only 22% of the population were covered by insurance policies, although coverage between oblasts is quite variable (Shiskin & Rozhdestvenskaya, 1995).

Secondly, the argument implicitly assumes that conditions external to the health sector have remained unchanged. This is clearly not the case. Private sector employment opportunities, for example, are expanding rapidly both in the medical and non-medical sectors. A bright young doctor now has a choice of working in the state sector, in private practice or even leaving medicine entirely and working for, for example, an international drugs company or as a translator. Similarly, allowing hospitals to admit private patients opens the possibility that providers may prefer to treat patients privately. Government will find that once opened, the Pandora's box of market opportunities will be difficult to close. It simply is not realistic to assume that additional money can reverse recent changes in the sector without more fundamental reform.

Thirdly, increasing funding without further reform suggests that the past pattern of medical provision was optimal. Yet there is ample evidence which suggests it was not. Although the system had positive features such as universal first-level care through feldsher stations, many other aspects of the system were flawed. The funding system placed excessive emphasis on inputs; resource flows were driven by normative-based staffing and bed allocations which were unrelated to size of population or other indicators of need. Too much emphasis was given to hospitalisation. The number of beds per capita exceeds most other countries (see Table 10.1) and the level of hospitalisation and length of stay once in hospital was also high. This meant that treating disease was a hospital-intensive process that placed great emphasis on specialist medicine rather than broad-based primary care. While the number of first-level ambulatory facilities was high, the relative level of funding was low. In recent years the collapse of many state farms has meant that funding has declined still further.

These technical inefficiencies in the system are compounded by a growing awareness of allocative inefficiencies through the use of treatments that are ineffective or cost ineffective. A recent conference in Almaty on quality in health care drew attention to two treatments that are routinely used: hyperbaric oxygenation and low frequency laser therapy (Zdrav Refom, 1996). Hyperbaric oxygenation, used to treat divers suffering the 'bends', has been used throughout the former Soviet bloc to treat liver diseases, such as viral hepatitis, poisonings and a wide variety of other illnesses. Low frequency laser therapy (not powerful enough to 'cut') is used to treat diseases such as rheumatoid arthritis and bronchial asthma. The evidence for both these treatments for many of their current uses is poor yet hospitals continue to purchase such technology in order to attract paying patients. There are many other similar examples.

Despite the problems with introducing medical insurance in depressed economies, a large number of the FSB countries have introduced insurance or written draft laws. By the middle of 1996 full systems were operating in Russia, Kazakstan, Estonia and Turkmenistan and pilot systems in Moldova and Kyrgyzstan. Laws were in preparation in Latvia, Lithuania and Uzbekistan. Most insurance laws are based on earmarked payroll taxes with contributions for the socially protected—children, elderly, registered unemployed and disabled—paid from the general budget. Turkmenistan has introduced a voluntary scheme, also aimed at the formal-sector employed, which pays for drugs and prostheses. The financial viability of this scheme is doubtful.

Despite reservations about the revenue reasons for introducing insurance, it would be a mistake to see this as the only or even main reason for introducing insurance. A key part of the introduction of insurance in Russia has been to create an internal market for purchasers as well as providers. The intention is to give patients a choice over which organisation buys health care on their behalf and induce health funds to compete.

10.2.2   Privatisation

Another feature of the reform process is the promotion of privatisation. Privatisation is encouraged for a variety of reasons. These include the dogmatic assertion that private sector is better than state, the pragmatic need to divest the state of an excessive number of facilities and a conviction that private sector realities will force providers to become more competitive and improve the quality of care.

Care is required in disentangling these reasons since there is a great danger that the worst aspects of private sector development are allowed to flourish while the best are not properly exploited for the benefit of the majority of the population.

The process of privatisation began in each country with the legalisation of private practice. This legitimised a practice that may well have been occurring in each country for some time. The most common forms of private practice are pharmacies and small private clinics. Often the latter are run by retired doctors or by employed doctors during their off-duty hours. Privatisation of hospitals is less common.

A danger is that unless the government can carefully control the process, user payments assume an increasing part in funding for health care so that providers reorient services to cater primarily for these patients. This 'creeping' privatisation or privatisation from within is illustrated well in the case of China where hospitals now find themselves obtaining much of their income from user payments. As a result they offer services that are profitable rather than medically necessary. There has been an enormous increase in the purchase and use of expensive scanning technology in the last 10 years, and it is reported that some insurance funds operate their scanners simply to boost billings to insurance funds. Countries in the FSB are not yet at this stage and can avoid this danger through appropriate policy. A problem in China has been that the state has allowed the sector to develop without really knowing how to regulate or monitor. It is essential that FSB countries define an appropriate role for the state so that regulation in these countries is effective.

10.2.3   Payment systems

Given the low level of medical wages it is not surprising that many countries have chosen to experiment with alternative methods of payment. The development of private and semi-private forms of provision has encouraged the use of fee for service methods of payment. This trend has been exacerbated by the development of medical insurance. Insurance funding and fee for service payment are believed to be linked—partly because both are aimed at providing individual rather than population-based care, and partly because established medical insurance systems in OECD countries often make heavy use of fee for service payment. An important role for policy advice is to show that this linkage need not be automatic.

The effects of various methods of payment are reviewed in detail in Chapter 5. The results of inappropriate payment systems have already been demonstrated in Eastern European countries such as the Czech Republic. In early insurance schemes in the former Soviet Union perverse incentives were also apparent. Estonian county funds found that they quickly ran out of money when a per diem system was introduced for paying for hospital treatment.

Similar effects are reported in the pilot systems introduced in Kazakstan. Some proposals have sought to overcome these perversities by introducing complex systems related to case-mix but introduced additional problems of monitoring and control.

10.2.4 Primary health care

There is a growing realisation that the system of ambulatory care in both rural and urban areas does not now form the basis of an effective system. There are a number of problems.

- The culture of the specialist means that primary physicians are not held in high esteem.
- No additional training is given to first-level doctors (paediatrician, gynaecologist and adult general physician) and patients often self-refer themselves to specialists.
- Self-referral is made easier because specialists work alongside generalists in the same polyclinic.
- Doctors move frequently.
- The system of territoriality means that each patient is assigned to a doctor—there is no choice.
- The prophylactic principle means that most of the population are visited on a regular basis. This is a resource-intensive system that is made less effective because practitioners often do not have the supplies or expertise to offer appropriate advice or care.
- Funding levels for primary care are low relative to secondary providers.
- There are few financial incentives to attract patients, provide preventive care or work in unpopular areas (although some incentives are given to all public workers for working in certain designated polluted areas).
- Since rural clinics are often underfunded, patients are often kept in hospital to receive follow-up care that could be performed in an out-patient setting.

Although the problems are quite well known, the solution is far less clear cut. Many countries are embracing the idea of a general-practitioner-led system funded on the basis of capitation. Yet this model has not yet been properly developed or tested for the specific conditions of transitional countries. Another option is to refine the idea of the polyclinic to incorporate certain financial incentives that reward performance while preserving the idea of an integrated service incorporating a variety of first-level providers. Fundholding, as introduced in the United Kingdom, is also being tested in countries such as Kyrgyzstan. A problem with these reforms is that the local community is often not involved in the changes and unaware even that change has occurred.

If reform is to have significant impact in this area it will be important to define what is meant by primary care. This will include defining the extent of involvement of community, patients, medical staff and the state institutions and in deciding on what type of service should be provided. The appropriate model of provision and system of incentives can then be decided.

10.3   AN APPROPRIATE ROLE FOR THE STATE

One of the most important policy issues to resolve is the appropriate role of the state in the reformed health care system. The analysis of markets and insurance in Chapters 1 and 2 suggested a number of roles including:

1.   Risk pooling funded through income-related contributions.
2.   Regulation of facilities, accreditation and planning.
3.   Purchasing medical care as an informed buyer.
4.   Managing the process of provision without necessarily controlling the delivery of medical care.

The transition to the market economy has made the role of the state much more uncertain. In the past the state provided funding for health care, 'purchased' care through direct disbursements to health facilities based on staff–bed related normatives, and managed hospitals, polyclinics and health centres. Overall strategic planning arose almost as a consequence of these other functions, although separate 'vertical' programmes were designed to target specific diseases. Funding in the system played a passive role, led by the level of inputs required to fulfil specific normatives.

In fact the question is made more complicated by the additional state institutions that are now involved in health care. These include the national administration (Ministry of Health), local oblast administrations, health insurance funds and state-owned providers. The question of state involvement is now twofold: what should it do and which institutions should undertake each role?

A list of the possible roles of the state is given in Table 10.2, together with a suggestion for their allocation between health administration, insurance fund and provider organisation.

Responsibility for *strategy* and *control* over the system properly lies with the state health administration at national and regional level. Historically, they were responsible for ensuring that funding was allocated in line with normatives, realigning normatives where appropriate and carrying out national vertical programmes. Introducing a greater degree of self-government into facilities and involving the private sector in provision means that there is less need for micro-management. The role in the reformed system is to provide

Table 10.2 Appropriate functions for the state?

	Health insurance fund	Health administration	Providers
Sources of funding			
Assessment and collection of contributions	✓	—	—
Actuarial comparison of long-run income and expenditure	✓	—	—
Expanding coverage	✓	—	—
Strategy and control			
Regulation of technology	—	✓	—
Pharmaceutical assessment and licensing	—	✓	—
Supplies procurement	—	✓	—
Payment for capital development/large equipment	?	?	—
Accreditation of facilities	—	✓	—
Licensing practitioners	—	✓	—
Planning (and executing) public health measures	—	✓	—
Regulation and procurement of expensive technologies	—	✓	—
Human resource planning	—	✓	—
Management training	?	?	—
Assisting providers to reduce costs and modify medical practice	?	?	—
Purchasing medical care			
Assessing health need	?	?	—
Assessing effectiveness of existing treatments	?	?	?
Developing protocols for treatment	?	?	?
Encouraging providers to modify practice	?	?	—
Negotiating with providers over cost savings	?	?	—
Payment of providers	✓	—	—
Monitoring treatment outcomes	?	?	—
Micro-management of medical facilities			
Staffing levels	—	?	✓
Bonuses	—	?	✓
Equipment purchases	—	?	✓
Use of facilities	—	?	✓
Type of services	✓	✓	✓

Note: ticks represent probable roles for respective organisations; question marks are possible roles.

information, monitor the entire system and provide services that the market is unable or unwilling to provide efficiently. This is entirely different from its historic role and will require radical readjustment of how these organisations operate. Discussions of these organisational questions are outside the scope of this book but are of considerable importance to all FSB countries.

The main unresolved issue is which organisation will take on responsibility for *purchasing* medical treatment. In theory insurance funds are well placed to fill this role since they are usually independent or quasi-independent of the ministry or oblast administration. Yet early results suggest that they are not carrying out this function adequately. There are a number of reasons for this which include:

- lack of knowledge of epidemiological data and how to interpret them;
- excessive concentration on payment for the medical treatment of individual patients rather than the population; and
- lack of training in purchasing skills.

Part of the problem is that often funds are only purchasing for a small proportion of the population and are not, therefore, required to take a population view. While funds are undertaking the payment of providers, sometimes using quite elaborate systems, other facets of purchasing are ignored. As argued in earlier chapters this can lead to services that are poorly planned and not responsive to population need.

It may not, therefore, be realistic to assume that insurance funds will become effective purchasers in the short term. In many ways this is unsurprising. Most of the health authorities in the UK had difficulty in becoming purchasers following the 1991 reforms, and purchasing capacity, in many areas, is still weak. Health funds in transition economies begin without any experience of public health or epidemiology, let alone health economics.

The absence of a purchaser in the reformed system is important given the tendency in many transition countries towards excess use of new technologies, over-prescription of medicines and use of treatments that are unproved or that may even be harmful. Any additional money obtained from insurance contributions could easily be swallowed up on these cost-ineffective practices unless a clearer direction is given to the process of change. Although normative financing was undoubtedly an imperfect allocation mechanism, it did at least ensure basic access to medical care for most of the population. At present no organisation is filling the gap left by the old system. The result could be to continue the process of 'creeping' privatisation and emphasis on inappropriate medical practice.

A middle course is for the purchasing functions to be shared between health administration, providers and insurance funds. The health administration could provide assistance to medical care facilities to restructure their services. This could be to develop management costing systems, help reorganise activity or providing information on more effective treatment regimes. One of the features of many of the centrally planned systems was that much data was collected but not used. Often data are quite comprehensive, competing in quantity and depth, if not quality, with the type of supply-side data collected in OECD countries. A task for new systems is to develop ways of using these data to enable hospitals to conduct evaluation of their services.

10.4   SUMMARY OF KEY POINTS FROM THE BOOK

What are the main lessons which emerge from this book for the operation of health systems, particularly in transitional countries?

Microeconomics highlights the importance of supply-induced demand as a feature of the health care market and the emphasis which should therefore be attached to incentives for suppliers. It stresses the efficiency benefits which can be reaped from competition or at least contestability, as long as these can be made to be compatible with other objectives, such as equity and cost containment. It also reinforces the desirability of freeing providers to manage resources more flexibly, while at the same time facilitating informed judgement by patients, by increasing the availability of information about services and their quality.

The review of *options for funding arrangements* argues that private user charges or private insurance are inadequate as the main funding source for the health sector, because of adverse selection, social externalities of health care, and uncertainty about demand. Any insurance system will also face problems of coverage, especially where large rural or informal sector workforces exist. The importance of institutional and economic development for the choice of systems of funding and payment is emphasised; the savings model of funding, for example, is presented as an option where systems are well developed and an individualistic culture is found. The level of competence of existing institutions will also affect their ability to take on new roles. Decentralisation, while offering potential advantages for day-to-day management, also makes it harder to redistribute resources between regions and makes supervision of the 'good behaviour' of local managers all the more important.

Economic evaluation is seen as a key tool in prioritising between health-related activities, given the overall resource constraints which all systems face. It assists in placing emphasis on outcomes, which so commonly are ignored in systems which generate their own internal goals (such as job preservation or professional enhancement). Even if not actively engaged in evaluations themselves, FSB health managers should understand the techniques used so as to be able to critically evaluate the results of trials published in the West and apply them as relevant in their local context. The need for careful methodology is emphasised, both in medical trials and the economic studies which may accompany them, so that the results are not misleading. The ongoing development of new medical technologies and the increasing pressure to buy them, both from commercial companies and the general public, will make use of economic evaluation increasingly important in FSB health systems over the next decades. Problems of funding also point to a possible move away from universalism and implicit rationing towards a more explicit rationing of public services, such as has occurred in other countries, like New Zealand and the USA.

The importance of the *purchasing function* is stressed, and this is of particular relevance to the FSB, where purchasing skills are lacking and the concept is a relatively new one. Given the information asymmetries in health care and the problem of moral hazard for consumers, combined with supply-induced demand, the purchaser's role is to modify demand and supply so that health priorities are followed and social welfare maximised. Although purchasers are rarely able to rethink health activities entirely, there is usually scope for benefits at the margin by reallocating from less to more cost-effective new activities. In the presence of a highly individualistic culture, however, this type of population-based planning is constrained by the emphasis on individual purchasing decisions.

It is unclear whether competition between purchasers brings benefits, particularly in less developed regions, because of the economies of scale and scope and the difficulty of judging purchaser performance. Regional monopsony may therefore be preferable in the FSB. Purchasers also need to maintain a balance between promoting partnerships with providers and promoting their long-term development and market stability, and promoting competition in the provider market.

Payments systems and their influence on the pattern of activities is a theme throughout the book. Clearly their operation will depend on the context, but in general terms capitation and volume contracts score highly, because they limit costs and are easy to establish and monitor. Most fee for service systems, by contrast, are costly to run and encourage cost escalation. Some, like DRGs, perform better in terms of cost control than the others, but these systems also tend to be more expensive to operate. Direct user payments by patients are unsuitable for basic treatments, but can be appropriate for extras and non-essential treatments as a way of raising additional resources and controlling demand.

Planning for providers and *option appraisal* recognise that providers often face few incentives to undertake fundamental change and that incentives may even discourage reform. However, in order to respond to increasing competition and as managerial scope is widened, it is important that they begin to develop a capability to plan their activities and respond to the reforms. As with purchasing and contracting, the ability to carry out increasingly sophisticated appraisal, costing and modelling exercises will require investment in staff training and information technology.

Contracting stresses the importance of agreeing activity levels so that purchaser and provider are protected against under- and over-trading. This may form the basic contract, which can later become more sophisticated, with allowance for case-mix, quality specifications, and possibly even outcome specifications.

Privatisation is fashionable in many countries, but this final chapter suggests that the term 'private' obscures more than it reveals, hiding the many dimensions that contribute towards an organisation behaving in a profit-maximising rather than state-controlled way. It is not so much ownership *per se* which will determine organisational behaviour, as how managerial control is exercised, how surplus is treated, what the balance of funding sources is, and the way in which the market is structured—such as price and quality regulation, the degree of competition, payment systems and the availability of information about performance.

The main question posed by this final chapter, and a theme running throughout the book, is what the role of the state will be in the reformed health sectors. The old historic role of the state has been challenged and has to adapt, but how state and private, central and local, profit and non-profit institutions can best interact to provide health care is not yet clear. What is important, however, is that comparative experience and a clear understanding of the local context and priorities, rather than dogma, guide decisions on structures and systems.

REFERENCES

Fraser, D. (1984) *The evolution of the British welfare state*. London: Macmillan. 2nd edition.

Hyde, G. (1974) *The Soviet health service*. London: Lawrence & Wishart.

Menzentseva, E. & Rimachevskaya, N. (1990) The Soviet country profile: health of the USSR population in the 70s and 80s—and approach to a comprehensive analysis. *Social Science and Medicine*, vol. 31, no. 8, pp. 867–877.

Rowland, D. & Telyukov, A.V. (1991) Soviet health care from two perspectives. *Health Affairs*, vol. 10, no. 3, pp. 71–86.

Shishkin, S. & Rozhdestvenskaya, J.A. (1995) *Social services provision under the transition (health care, education, culture)*. Paper for the Institute for the Economy in Transition, Moscow.

Social Indicators of Development. 1995. Washington, DC: World Bank.

World Development Report 1996: From plan to market. Washington, DC: World Bank.

Zdrav Refom (1996) Effectiveness in health care: laser therapy and hyperbaric oxygen, in conference notes for *National Conference on Assuring Quality of Care*, Almaty, Kazakstan, 15–16 May.

GLOSSARY

Acceptability Degree to which a service meets the cultural needs and standards of a community. This in turn will affect utilisation of that service.

Accessibility Extent to which a service is easy to use for its intended clients. This will depend on a number of factors, such as its costs (see *affordability*), its distance from them, the way in which services are organised, etc.

Adverse selection A situation where individuals are able to purchase insurance at rates which are below actuarially fair rates, because information known to them is not available to insurers (*asymmetric information*).

Affordability Extent to which the intended clients of a service can pay for it. This will depend on their income distribution, the cost of services and the financing mechanism (e.g. whether risks are pooled; whether exemptions exist for the low-paid etc.)

Agency relationship A situation in which one person (agent) makes decisions on behalf of another person (principal).

Annuitisation/annualisation Process by which a *capital cost* is converted into an annual cost, by dividing the overall cost by the number of expected life years, and adjusting for the *discount rate*.

Asymmetric information Situations in which the parties on the opposite sides of a transaction have differing amounts of relevant information.

Audit Originally the process by which the probity of operations and activities of an organisation was examined (internal audit) and a report on the annual accounts produced (external audit). Now used more widely, e.g. clinical audit evaluates the effectiveness of clinical activities; management audit the effectiveness and efficiency of organisational and management arrangements etc.

Average cost Total cost represents the sum of all *fixed costs* and *variable costs*. Average cost equals total cost divided by the quantity of output

Average length of stay (ALOS) The average number of days a patient stays in hospital.

Bed occupancy   The number of beds occupied by patients at a particular time, expressed as a percentage of available beds or as the number of days each bed is occupied each year.

Bed turnover   The average number of patients using each bed in a given period, such as a year.

Bias   Deviation of results or inferences from the truth, or processes leading to such deviation. Any trend in the collection, analysis, interpretation, publication, or review of data that can lead to conclusions that are systematically different from the truth.

Capital costs   Expenditure on goods which last longer than one year, such as investment in equipment or infrastructure.

Capitation   A method of reimbursement under which a provider is paid a fixed amount per person regardless of the volume of services rendered.

Case fatality rate (CFR)   The proportion of cases of a specific condition which are fatal within a specified time. CFR (given as %) = no. of deaths from a disease in a given period divided by no. of diagnosed cases of that disease in the same period.

Case-mix   A measure of the assortment of patient cases treated by a given hospital, indicating the degree of complexity of the cases.

Coinsurance (rate)   The share of costs which are paid by the beneficiary of a health policy (often after some *deductible*).

Command economy   Where the government decides how much of each good should be produced, how and for whom. The opposite to the '*free market*' paradigm, in which prices are set purely by the force of supply and demand. In reality, though, few economies operate in either of these two pure ways: more common are planned markets, regulated markets or managed markets, with varying degrees of involvement of government in market operations and outcomes.

Complements   Goods which are normally consumed together, so that an increase in the price of one will lead to a decrease in demand for the other.

Compounding   The process by which a sum of money now is given its future value, calculated according to the number of years and the annual discount rate.

Compulsory health insurance   Health insurance under an obligatory public scheme. Payment for such an insurance amounts to a tax. Employers may have to pay contributions on behalf of their employees. Contributions are usually income-related. Compulsory health insurance is usually, but not always, administered by a public body.

Contingent valuation   A method of eliciting the value set by individuals on such goods as life itself. A variety of methods have been developed to convert such *intangible* benefits or costs into monetary figures, in order to compare with other possible activities.

Contracts   The basis for agreement on what services should be provided to patients, which may include a specification of quality. **Block contracts** (or capitation contracts in a primary care setting) specify which services are to be provided, and to whom, and the total payment to be made, but without fixing the volume of services to be delivered. **Cost and volume contracts** specify the type and level of services required by the purchaser. If fewer services are provided, some of the payment can be withheld. On the other hand, if levels are exceeded, additional payments will be made to providers, according to some pre-agreed scale. **Cost per case contracts** set the cost of specific treatments only, with no limits on total payments or eventual volume of services.

Copayment   Amounts paid by the insurance beneficiary as a result of *coinsurance* and *deductibles*.

Cost–benefit analysis (CBA)   A method of comparing the monetary value of all benefits of a social project with all costs of that project.

Cost control   Ability to limit the resources used in a particular service or sector. This is one of the criteria frequently used to judge health sector performance (along with *efficiency*, *equity*, *acceptability* etc.)

Cost-effectiveness analysis (CEA)   A method of comparing the costs of a social project with the benefits, measured in terms of a social objective. Something which is cost effective achieves relatively high gains for relatively low costs, compared with other possible ways of achieving that goal.

Cost-sharing   Methods of financing health care which require some direct payments for services by patients. (See also *copayment*.)

Cost–utility analysis (CUA)   A method of comparing the costs of a social project with the benefits, measured in terms of an overall index of both quantity and quality of life gained (see *QALY*). This avoids the need to convert social benefits into monetary terms, but at the same time allows for comparisons between programmes with differing social objectives. However, collecting reliable information on changes to quality of life is relatively difficult.

Cream skimming   Practice by which insurers or doctors discourage patients with expensive needs from joining their scheme or practice in order to protect their profit margins. Even if illegal, it can be achieved by subtle means such as having poor access to facilities for the elderly or disabled.

Deductible   The amount of health care charges for which a beneficiary is responsible before the insurer begins payment.

Demand   The quantity of a good purchased at any given price.

Depreciation   The change in the value of a good over time, due to deteriorating physical characteristics or technical obsolescence.

Diagnosis-related groups (DRGs)   A set of case types established under the *prospective payment system* (*PPS*) identifying patients with similar conditions and processes of care. Used for setting charges for different health care interventions.

Direct costs   This term is used slightly differently in different contexts. In allocating costs in hospitals, direct costs are the costs which are incurred by patient departments (producing final outcomes), as opposed to the paraclinic, support and overhead departments (which produce intermediary goods). In evaluations, however, the distinction is being made between costs which are actually paid by the health service or patients, as opposed to the opportunity costs of time and production lost as a result of treatment (termed *indirect costs*), which are also real but are often omitted from consideration.

Discounting/discount rate   The process of converting sums to be received at a future date to a present value. The interest rate which is used is called the discount rate.

Economies of scale   Situations in which the *long run* average costs of a firm are declining as output is increasing.

Economies of scope   Situations in which a firm can jointly produce two or more goods more cheaply than under separate production of the goods.

Effectiveness   The extent to which a specific intervention, procedure, regimen or service, when deployed in the field, does what it is intended to do for a defined population.

Efficacy   The extent to which a specific intervention, procedure, regimen, or service produces a beneficial result under ideal conditions. Ideally, the determination of efficacy is based on the results of a *randomised controlled trial*.

Efficiency   When the firm produces the maximum possible sustained output from a given set of inputs this is known as **technical efficiency**. This idea is distinguished from **allocative efficiency**, in which either inputs or outputs are put to their best possible uses in the economy so that no further gains in output or welfare are possible.

Elasticity Percentage change in some dependent variable (e.g. quantity demanded) resulting from a 1% change in some independent variable (e.g. price). Elasticities which exceed one in absolute value are considered elastic; elasticities less than one are inelastic.

Epidemiology Study of the distribution and determinants of disease in human populations.

Equilibrium price (quantity) The price (quantity) at which the quantity demanded and quantity supplied are equal.

Equity At its most general, equity means being fair or just. How to judge that is subjective and controversial, and part of the policy-maker's mandate rather than the economist's. However, a common understanding is that everyone should have geographical and financial access to available resources in health care.

Essential drugs A policy initiative to ensure that a minimal number of effective drugs is available to treat priority health problems at a cost which can be afforded by the community. A related aim is to save the resources used by prescribing more expensive or even unnecessary drugs.

Exemptions Rules allowing certain groups in society (the socially disadvantaged, generally) not to pay charges or insurance premia. The difficulty lies in defining which categories should be exempt and in monitoring the system.

Externality A case in which a consumer (producer) affects the utility (costs) of another consumer (producer) through actions which lie outside the price system.

Factors of production The inputs which are required to produce any good. At a general level, these are divided into labour, land and capital (both finance and equipment).

Fee for service (FFS) A method of payment under which the provider is paid for each procedure or service that is provided to a patient.

Feldsher A rural paramedic, with a similar role to an assistant doctor in developing countries. Receives basic nurse training and further training in diagnosis and referral.

Firm Any entity that transforms inputs into some product or service that is sold in the marketplace.

Fixed costs (TFC and AFC) Costs which do not vary with output. They are expressed either as total fixed cost (TFC) or average fixed cost (AFC).

Free markets A term used to denote an economy in which government plays little role in production and distribution of goods. It is misleading to the extent that all markets require rules and regulations to function effectively, and in that sense cannot be totally 'free'. (See also *command economy*.)

General practitioner (GP) A UK term, meaning a general doctor, or family doctor, who is the first point of contact with health services for all non-emergency cases. GPs in the UK are self-employed but contracted by the government to provide a range of basic diagnostic, preventive and curative services. They refer cases as appropriate to hospital-based specialists. (See *GP fundholder*.)

Global budget An aggregate cash sum, fixed in advance (usually for one year), intended to cover the total costs of a service, whatever the eventual workload.

Good Economic term, meaning a commodity whose consumption provides utility for individuals.

GP fundholder A UK general practitioner practice with a budget which includes purchase of a range of hospital in-patient and out-patient and other services. Now being expanded to 'total fundholding', so that GPs can purchase the full range of referral services.

Gross National Product (GNP)/Gross Domestic Product (GDP) GNP is the current value of all final goods and services produced by a country during a year. GDP is a closely related measure which includes the value associated only with domestic factors of production.

Health Can be defined narrowly as the absence of illness, or more broadly as the 'state of complete physical, mental and social well-being', as the WHO Constitution declares.

Health care Goods and services used as inputs to produce health. In some analyses, one's own time and knowledge used to maintain and promote health are considered in addition to conventional health care inputs.

Health maintenance organisation (HMO) An organisation which, in return for a prepaid premium, provides an enrollee with comprehensive health benefits for a given period of time.

Health status Measures of the physical and emotional well-being of an individual or a defined population. (See also *morbidity rate* and *mortality rate*.)

Hotel costs The costs of food, heating, maintenance etc. for keeping a patient in hospital, excluding all medical and treatment costs.

Human capital The durable labour skills obtained by investment in oneself through education, training, health and so forth.

Human capital approach Method of valuing lives gained in terms of the discounted productive capacity of the patients treated.

Incentives Systems which reward and therefore tend to encourage certain types of activity.

Income effect The effect on quantity demanded that results from the change in real income associated with a relative change in the price of the good or service under study. (See also *substitution effect*.)

Income elasticity of demand/supply Percentage change in quantity demanded (supplied) resulting from a 1% change in income. (See also *elasticity*.)

Indirect costs Usually used in economic evaluation, to indicate the opportunity costs of production or leisure time lost in order to undergo treatment. Distinguished from *direct costs* and *intangible costs*.

Infant mortality rate (IMR) The ratio of the number of deaths in infants one year or less during a year, divided by the number of live births during the year.

Inferior good A good or service for which demand decreases as income increases. (See also *normal* and *superior goods*.)

In-patient A patient who has been admitted to hospital and is occupying a bed in an in-patient department.

Intangible costs Usually used in economic evaluation, to indicate features like pain, anxiety or grief, which are very important, but hard to measure or value in monetary terms.

International Classification of Disease (ICD) Classification of conditions and groups of conditions by an international group of experts who advise the World Health Organisation. The WHO publishes the complete list periodically.

Long run A period of time sufficient to permit a firm to vary all factors of production. (See also *short run*.)

Luxury good A good with a *price elasticity* of greater than one, such that demand is highly responsive to price changes. (See also *necessity*.)

Macroeconomics Looking at the operation of the economy as a whole.

Managed care A term encompassing a broad set of actions which a firm or insurer establishes to reduce costs.

Marginal Produced by an increase of one unit.

Marginal cost The increase in total cost resulting from a one unit increase in output.

Marginal utility   The extra utility gained from consuming one more unit of a good, holding others constant. Utility is a measure of the satisfaction from consuming goods.

Market structure   How an industry is organised in terms of the number and distribution of firms and how firms compete among themselves.

Meta-analysis   Using statistical methods to combine the results of different studies. It involves qualitative measures to select the studies to be used, and quantitative methdods in combining them to produce statistically significant results. It runs the risk of several biases.

Microeconomics   Looking at interactions in a specific market or for a specific good.

Monopoly   Literally: single seller. Situation in which a firm faces a negatively sloped demand curve. In a pure monopoly, there is no other firm which produces a close substitute for the firm's product. Thus the demand curve facing the monopolist is the market demand curve.

Monopoly profit (rent)   The return over and above a normal profit resulting from monopoly power.

Monopsony   Literally: single buyer. Situation in which a firm faces a positively sloped supply curve in the product or factor market.

Moral hazard   An insurance term. Where services are not paid for directly by individuals, they may take risks or act in a way which increases the demand for health services. It is in insurers' interests to create disincentives to such behaviour (such as *copayments* or risk-rated *premia*).

Morbidity rate   The rate of incidence of disease in a particular population.

Mortality rate   The death rate for a particular population. The crude death rate is the ratio of deaths during a year divided by mid-year population. Because age is so important, the age-adjusted mortality rate is a measure which takes into account a population's age distribution.

Necessity   A good whose consumption does not vary greatly with changes in price—i.e. a good with a *price elasticity of demand* of less than one.

Needs   What a person requires in terms of health care. Judged subjectively this is often called WANTS, to distinguish it from an objective judgement about appropriate treatment. Commonly needs are judged by a professional, which introduces a different kind of bias. These are distinguished from what is actually purchased, which is DEMAND.

Nominal value   The money value measured in current dollars. (See also *real value*.)

Normal good   A good or service for which demand increases in proportion as income increases. (See also *inferior* and *superior goods*.)

Oblast   A region in the former Soviet Union.

Opportunity cost   The value of the best alternative which is forgone in order to get or produce more of the commodity under consideration.

Optimality   A productive arrangement which produces the greatest possible welfare for a given set of inputs.

Outcome   The effect on health status of a health care intervention, or lack of intervention.

Out-patient   A patient attending for treatment or a consultation, but not staying overnight in a hospital.

Payroll taxes   Taxes which are specifically earmarked for a sector, like health. Distinguished from *social insurance* because entitlement is not limited to those who have paid contributions.

Perfect competition   A market structure in which there are (1) numerous buyers and sellers, (2) perfect information, (3) free entry and exit, and (4) a homogeneous product.

Polyclinic   In the former Soviet Union, these are normally the first point of contact for patients with the health services. They provide first-level care and, in many cases, specialist out-patient services too.

Premium   Payment for voluntary insurance. Premiums may be community rated (averaged across a group of individuals) or risk rated (tailored to the claims experience or actuarial risk of each individual).

Price elasticity of demand/supply   Percentage change in quantity demanded (supplied) resulting from a 1% change in price. (See also *elasticity*.)

Price index   Expresses the current prices of a group of goods relative to the prices of these goods in a base year. A price index, often used to convert *nominal values* (i.e. current prices) to *real values*, shows how much prices of those goods have changed since the base year.

Primary care   In a system with a gatekeeper, all initial (non-emergency) consultations with doctors, nurses or other health staff are termed primary care, as opposed to *secondary care* or referral services. In systems with direct access to specialists, the distinction is usually based on facilities, with polyclinics, for example, providing primary care and hospitals secondary care. (See also *primary health care*.)

Primary health care (PHC)   According to WHO, PHC is essential health care made accessible at a cost which the country and community can afford, with methods that are practical, scientifically sound and socially acceptable. It is a normative concept, implying access for all, community participation and the importance of prevention and a multi-sectoral approach to the production of health.

Prioritisation   Deciding the relative importance attached to alternative goals or activities in a given setting. It is often connected with resource shortages and the need to *ration* care.

Productivity   The output produced for a given input.

Progressive (tax)   Tax or other form of financing in which the percentage of the contribution to be paid rises with rising income levels. (See *regressive*.)

Prospective payment system (PPS)   The method of hospital reimbursement used by Medicare in the US from 1983 under which hospitals were reimbursed a fixed amount for each patient treated, according to their *diagnosis-related groups (DRGs)*.

Provider   An organisation which provides health care, such as a primary care doctor or a hospital, and sells its services to purchasers.

Public good (pure)   A good (e.g. national defence) that no one can be prevented from consuming (non-excludable), and that can be consumed by one person without depleting it for another (non-rival). The marginal cost of providing the good to another consumer is zero.

Purchaser   A health care body which assesses the needs of a defined population and buys services to meet those needs from providers.

QALY   Quality-adjusted life year—a measure of health gain which aims to measure life years added but also the quality of life which is achieved in those years. This is one measure used in *cost–utility analysis*. Another is the DALY (disability-adjusted life year, developed by the World Bank and WHO)—a narrower definition, but easier to measure.

Randomised controlled trial (RCT)   A trial to establish the efficacy of a given medical treatment, in which patients are identified according to strict eligibility criteria and randomly allocated to a treatment or control group; the assessors of outcomes are also usually 'blind'—i.e. unaware of which group each patient belongs to. The aim of these procedures is to remove biases and increase the accuracy of the trial results.

Rationing   Restricting supply of services according to implicit or explicit criteria, where demand exceeds supply. It implies the absence of fully functioning market mechanisms to link demand with supply.

Rayon   A district in the former Soviet Union.

Real value   Monetary values that are adjusted for changes in the general level of priccs relative to some arbitrarily selected base year. (See also *nominal value*.)

Recurrent expenditure   Expenditure which has to be incurred during each budget period, such as on salaries, drugs, supplies, provision and maintenance.

Regressive (tax)   Form of tax or other financing in which the proportion of income paid falls with rising income levels.

Regulation   Government intervention in the functioning of markets. Can be of a 'market-enhancing' type, designed to encourage competition between firms, or a 'market-replacing' type, with the state intervening directly in production and distribution (see *command economy*).

Risk aversion   The degree to which a certain income is preferred to a risky alternative with the same expected income.

Secondary care   Care provided by medical specialists, usually in a hospital setting (see *primary care*), but also some specialist services provided in the community.

Semi-variable costs   Costs which increase as output increases, but unevenly, as certain levels of output are reached.

Sensitivity analysis   Testing how a result might change if key variables are altered. Relevant variables to test are ones where there is uncertainty about their expected value. A range of realistic values is then drawn up, and the end result recalculated to see whether its broad conclusion would be altered if those values were realised.

Shadow prices   Market prices adjusted for distortions, for example in the price which can be charged for the good, the value of foreign currency, the cost of labour or cost of capital in a given sector or economy. Shadow prices are supposed to reflect more accurately the opportunity cost of the good being produced.

Short run   Situations in which the firm is not able to vary all its inputs. There is at least one factor of production that is fixed. (See also *long run*.)

Social insurance   Government insurance programmes in which eligibility and premiums are not determined by the practices common to private insurance contracts. Premiums are often subsidised and there are typically redistributions from some segments of the population to others.

Standardised mortality ratio (SMR)   The number of deaths in a given year as a percentage of those expected. The expected number is a standard mortality adjusted for age and sex.

Substitutes   Substitutes in consumption are goods that satisfy the same wants (e.g. beef and chicken) so that an increase in the price of one will increase the demand for the other. Substitutes in production are alternative goods which a firm can produce (e.g. corn and soybeans for a farmer) so that an increase in the price of one will lead to a decrease in the supply of another.

Substitution effect   The change in quantity demanded resulting from a relative change in commodity prices, holding real income constant. (See also *income effect*.)

Superior good   A good or service for which demand increases as income increases. (See also *inferior good*.)

Supplier-induced demand (SID)   The change in demand associated with the discretionary influence of providers, especially doctors, over their patients. Demand that is partly influenced by the self-interest of providers rather than solely by patient interests.

SWOT analysis   A management tool for examining the internal performance of a firm and its response to external developments. The focus is on its current strengths and weaknesses, and the opportunities and threats provided by the environment.

Third-party payment   Refers to situations where the first party (patient) does not pay directly for the activities of the second party (providers), but this is done through a private insurer, sickness fund or government agency (third party). This set-up will affect the quantity of the service demanded and supplied.

Time preference   The degree to which a sum, say $1, is worth more now than it would be in one year (excluding the issues of inflation or uncertainty).

Transaction costs   The costs which are incurred by the process of negotiating between buyer and seller—for example, the cost of collecting information about products, drawing up contracts, negotiating prices etc. These reduce the profitability of doing business in that market.

Transitional economy   Term used to describe economies which used to be run on *command* lines, but which are now giving an increased role to market forces. As the term implies, they are still in the process of reform, and not yet fully established market economies.

Treatment protocol   Written guidelines for the management of a given condition, specifying actions to be taken by different professionals and, where appropriate, the patient. These are intended to encourage continuity of care between different professionals involved in a case, clearer communication with the patient, and consistent application of 'best practice' by the professionals.

User charges   Direct payment for services by patients, though not necessarily covering the full costs of that service. These are often introduced to supplement public finance for health services which used to be free. Charges can be officially sanctioned and their levels controlled, but commonly they develop informally and vary between facilities and even members of staff.

Utilisation   Use of capacity, often measured as an average over a period (e.g. bed occupancy, or theatre usage).

Utilitarian   Adopting the philosophy developed by Jeremy Bentham in the nineteenth century, which suggested as an overall social goal 'the greatest happiness of the greatest number'.

Utility   Economic term indicating the welfare gained by individuals through consumption. The assumption is that individuals 'maximise utility', so that, in general, more consumption is better than less, other things being equal.

Variable costs   Costs associated with factor(s) of production which change in quantity according to the quantity of output. Often expressed as a total variable cost (TVC) or average variable cost (AVC).

Voluntary health insurance   Health insurance which is taken up and paid for at the discretion of individuals (whether directly or via their employers). It can be offered by a public or private company.

Weighted capitation   Sum of money provided for each resident in a particular locality. The three main factors commonly reflected in the formula are: age structure of the population; its morbidity; and the relative cost of providing services.

World Health Organisation (WHO)   United Nations organisation, based in Geneva, responsible for promotion of health throughout the world.

SOURCES

Follard, S., Goodman, A. & Stano, M. (1993) *The economics of health and health care*. New York: Macmillan.

Last, J.M. (1988) *A dictionary of epidemiology*. Oxford: Oxford University Press for IEA. 2nd edition.

NHS Handbook 1995/6. 10th edn. JMH Publishing for NAHAT.

INDEX

Note: Page references in *italics* refer to Figures; those in **bold** refer to Tables

Index compiled by Annette Musker